29 AGAIN

&

Other Cancer-Fighting Stories

by

Mark Barkawitz

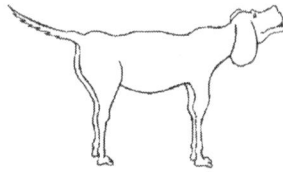

Edited

by

Nick Barkawitz

Cover Photo - Curaphotography - Big Stock

Cover Design - RomCon

For those who treat and seek to cure,
particularly Dr. Eddie Hu, Dr. Myo Htut,
Dr. Luciano Gomez, & Dr. Rahul Jandial.
Thanks, All.

To My Old Friend Bobby,

Stay healthy, Bro!
Walk, bike, swim, lift.
What else do you have to do?

Mark Burt   10/15

CONTENTS

INTRODUCTION

There are few things like a cancer diagnosis to throw your whole world into turmoil. It used to be a certain death sentence. But now, doctors are able to save two-out-of-three cancer patients. And those numbers will continue to improve in the foreseeable future.

A few of these stories were written before my own diagnosis, but most are a direct result of it, recounting my treatment and experiences as a patient in the rapidly-improving world of 21st century medicine. All are creatively factual; a few are fictionally hopeful. Cancer used to have a way of writing its own stories. But now in many cases, doctors have the tools to rewrite the endings.

One day in the middle of all this, my wife asked me: "How come you're always making jokes about your condition?" To which I replied: "Gallows humor." And similarly, an editor friend who published a few of the stories in my first-person narrative wrote to me: "How you manage to inject humor and affecting inspiration into such trial by fire circumstances is part of your innate gift." I hope others will think so, too, and be encouraged.

50% of all proceeds from this book
will be donated to City of Hope.

ROSE and AL

Back when I was in college, the walls of our duplex were thin plaster, so I was again awakened by my neighbor Al's coughing and hacking in the adjoining bedroom of the apartment next door. Al was 71 or 84 or 67, depending on how he felt each time I asked him. He'd had lung cancer for seventeen years. His first doctor had given him a year to live. Six months later, the doctor died. Since then, Al had buried two more doctors and a couple wives (according to his count), and still smoked two-packs-a-day—Camels, no filters.

But his current wife Rose—in her late fifties and *still a pup* as Al put it—had confirmed his getting worse of late. She was probably out on the couch in the living room, "Tryin' ta get some sleep!"

Between hacks, Al was probably lighting-up another smoke. I turned over in bed and pulled the pillow over my ear. But it was hard getting back to sleep.

1

MARK BARKAWITZ

BETTER BOOBS

"How do you like my new boob, Mike?" Kelly smiled as I approached her on the front porch of her Sierra Madre cottage. She stuck her left one forward for me to inspect. It was impossible to detect any difference under her sweater and bra.

"Looks good to me." I was a painting contractor, mostly residential, so I tended to work with a lot of women in their homes. I drank a lot of coffee and tended to talk a lot, too. Sometimes, they confided in me. Last year, just as I was putting the finishing touches on Kelly's kitchen remodel, she was diagnosed with breast cancer. Her sister had died a few years earlier of the same cancer. Kelly had gone through a lot in the year since I'd seen her: mastectomy, chemo, radiation, recovery, and finally—her new boob. We hugged.

"You look good, Kid."

"Thanks. I feel good." She smiled again. "Gary likes it, too." Gary was her husband.

I laughed. I did that a lot, too. We went inside. She poured me a cup of coffee. I leaned against the counter,

3

sipped her strong, hot brew, and we gabbed for the next hour or so about everything except cancer. We finally got around to scheduling a starting date for some touch-ups around the house. I put my empty coffee cup in her sink.

"You have another job to go to today?" she asked.

"Yep. Or I'd let you feed me, too." She was a good cook. We both laughed. Kelly did that a lot, too. Probably why we got along so well.

"Next time," she said.

We hugged goodbye and I hurried out to my truck, where I'd left my cellphone on the seat. One missed call. I recognized the number; it was Waters', my next job. I called back.

"Haylo?" It was the housekeeper's voice.

"Mariela?"

"*Si*. Is that you, Mikey?"

"*Si*."

"Mar-rgo wants to know if you still coming today?" Margo Waters was the homeowner. It had been a few months since I'd last worked at the Waters' Castle, as I called it. It was an old, 2½-story, 28-room, concrete-walled, multi-million-dollar mansion on Pasadena's west side above the Arroyo Seco and overlooking the Rose Bowl. I'd painted one room seven years ago and had worked there doing odd jobs on-and-off ever since.

"I'm on my way. Did you miss me?"

"Oh, *si*. You so nice. You always help Mariela."

I carried groceries up the back stairs for her; nothing any gentleman wouldn't do for a lady. No big deal.

"I have sooprise," she said.

"For me?"

"No, ees not for you. But ees sooprise."

Fifteen minutes later, I turned into the long driveway that led back to the castle. I parked, grabbed a few hand tools I might need from the toolbox in the truck bed, and headed up the back stairway. Through the row of kitchen windows on the landing, I saw Mariela inside at the sink. I knocked on the door, but opened it myself.

"Morning."

"Hi, Mikey. Coffee ees in microwave for you." She continued to wash dishes in the sink. "Mar-rgo go to gym. Leave note for you." Without turning towards me, she indicated with a nod that it was on the island.

I turned on the microwave, checked the note. I recognized Margo's handwriting:

-fix latch on cab in Butler's Pantry

-paint walls in Guest Room

"Margo's sister went home?"

"*Si*."

"How is she?"

Mariela shook her head. "Ees no good. Berry sick."

I nodded. Margo's sister was currently going through what Kelly had gone through last year. But her sister had been pregnant at the time the cancer was discovered, which had delayed and complicated her treatment and the cancer had spread. The oven dinged. I took out the cup, sipped the steamy coffee, went back to the list:

-replace all burnt-out light bulbs

-move potted trees from east patio to west patio

-assemble automatic cat box

"'Automatic cat box?'"

"*Si.* Mar-rgo get a new kitty."

"Really?" In all the time I'd worked in the castle, the Waters had never had a pet. From under the island, a black paw reached out for my shoelace. I put down the cup, got down on one knee and bent low. Yellow-green, almond-shaped eyes stared back at me from the jet-black face of a young feline—too old to be a kitten, too young to be a cat—perched like a sphinx, ready to pounce. "Hey, there." I reached in to pet its head between ears pointed upright. "What's its name?"

"Hair-rball."

"'Hairball?' That's funny. How you doing, Hairball?" It purred gently. Then I noticed each nail on its front paws was coated with some kind of clear, plastic sheath. I took its paw in my hand to inspect it more closely. "What the heck?"

Still at the sink, Mariela looked down. "Ees so kitty won't scratch furniture."

"You're kidding?" I ran my fingers across the floor in front of Hairball, who reached out to spoke my hand with its paw. The soft, acrylic sheaths kept its fingernails from digging into the skin on the back of my hand. I had to laugh. "What will they think of next?" Then I remembered the list—"*-assemble automatic cat box*"—and figured I'd find out soon enough.

"How's you knee?" Mariela asked.

"Not bad. Rehab took a while, but I'm back up to five or six miles a run now." I'd hurt it last summer. Didn't know how. Just woke up one morning and out of nowhere the darn thing was swollen like a volleyball. I sipped the coffee and found the loose latch in the adjoining pantry, took the Phillips screwdriver from the back pocket of my Levis, and carefully tightened the guilty, loose screw heads. "How's your back?" I asked through the doorway.

"Oh, ees *bueno*. I'm so glad. I tell Mar-rgo ees no more heavy lifting." She had been wearing a brace because of a lower back strain, but it was hard to tell under her baggy sweatshirt if she were still wearing it. She dried her hands on the dishtowel, turned to me with a funny, conspiratorial sort of look on her face. "You remember what we talk about last time you are here?"

I thought back.

"Come on." She prodded me: "You remember." She smiled and winked.

"Oh." I did suddenly remember—breast implants. Mariela had lost thirty pounds over the last year but had confessed to being unhappy with how the weight-loss had left her breasts, so she had consulted a plastic surgeon in the San Fernando Valley. I glanced down slightly, but the loose-fitting sweatshirt hid any clear indication. So risking a *faux pas*, I was compelled to ask uneasily: "Did you do it?"

She pursed her lips and nodded.

"Really?" I looked again, more closely. "Obviously, you didn't opt for the Ds." Her husband's suggestion, as I remembered.

"No." She shook her head. "Ees a full C."

"Ah-h. 'A full C.'"

"You want to see?"

"What?"

"Come on. I show you." She walked ahead of me farther into the house. I followed—What else could I do?—through the dining room, where from a wall-sized painting the luminous faces of Renaissance men and women stared judgmentally down at me, into a small hallway, where she closed the doors at both ends. She turned to me and pulled up the baggy sweatshirt, under which firm, twin mounds—like cantaloupe halves—were wrapped snuggly by a cotton crop top.

"Oh." I couldn't help staring, but didn't figure it rude in this instance anyway.

"Ees no bra," she stated proudly.

"'No, bra?' You're kidding?"

She shook her head. "No. Ees too sensitive." She covered them up again, smiled again. "Eh?"

"To quote my favorite sitcom: 'They're spectacular.' Good for you. Good for your husband, too," I kidded.

"Oh, he crazy now. He keep asking doctor: 'How soon? How soon?'"

"So you haven't tried them out yet?"

"No, no, no." She wagged her index finger like a mother playfully instructing a child. "Ees too sensitive. Doctor say ees okay for Saturday night."

"Really?" I smiled, thinking of her husband. "This Saturday?"

She nodded, wagged her finger at me again. "Doan you tell no one. Ees secret. No want Mar-rgo to know. I tell her I have back surgery. Take two weeks off. Thees morning she look over while I cook. But I no tell her."

"Yeah, she might get ticked-off now that her house-keeper has better boobs." We both laughed.

A door closed with a thud from the kitchen end of the house.

"Ees Mar-rgo. I go now." She hurried out the doorway towards the kitchen. I knew she'd clean-up my half-finished coffee cup on the way.

I went the other direction, up the stairs to the guest room, where the pillows were perfectly arranged on the bed and the bedspread was pulled snuggly across the mattress—not a wrinkle to indicate a human being had ever slept there. The blue walls didn't really need patching or painting, but Margo quite often changed colors on a whim—sometimes her own, sometimes her interior decorator's. A paint chip card was scotch-taped to the wall; the soft yellow color was named: "Morning." I took the flat-head screwdriver from my back pocket and began removing the brass faceplates, putting them all together in an empty wastebasket. A few minutes later, Margo poked her head in the room. "Hi, Mike."

"Hey, Margo. How goes it?"

"Okay." But she sounded weary, not convincing. She wore a designer work-out jacket and pants. She had recently turned forty, but was quite fit and attractive. A personal trainer at the gym and the Wonder bra under her little, white T-shirt helped.

"Sister moved back home. Huh?"

She nodded. "Yeah. She and the kids left last week." They had been staying with Margo during her sister's treatment at the USC-Norris Cancer Center.

"How is she?"

She shrugged her shoulders. "It's too early to tell." Sounding like a doctor, she educated me on the billions of cancer cells that had made up the multiple tumors that had forced the removal of both breasts, then maximum chemo and radiation treatments. Her sister's hair had fallen out. She had lost 25 pounds.

Trying to give Margo some hope, I told her about Kelly and her new boob.

"That's nice. But it won't save your friend if the cancer comes back."

I got more stuff from the truck, covered the furniture with plastic and the carpet with drop-cloths. I'd paint the walls tomorrow. Change-out the lights and assemble the automatic cat box, too. Today, tomorrow? What the heck did it matter? I didn't see Margo or Mariela on my way out. But it was a big house; you could get lost. So in the kitchen, I wrote a note on the island to let them know I'd be back first thing tomorrow. From under the island, the black paw reached out for my pant leg, but its prophylactic nails couldn't hook me.

No one was home when I got there, so I put on my running shorts and shoes, covered my bare skin with sunscreen, pulled down the bill of my cap, and went for a run. A long run. A very long run. But the melancholy stayed with me like a dog on a leash—*if the cancer comes back.* By the time I got home, it was nearly dark and my wife's car was parked behind my truck in the driveway. My knee ached again, as I climbed our front porch steps. My daughter let me in. She was thirteen and wearing a bra now. They ought to make those darn things cancer-proof. That'd be a Wonder bra!

"Hi, Dad. How was your run?"

"I don't know."

She screwed up her face. "You're so weird."

"Where's your brother?"

"At the Mall with Valerie." My son was seventeen. Valerie was his girlfriend. She drove a hot-yellow, convertible Mustang, which made my wife uneasy. "Mom's in the kitchen."

But I had already smelled our dinner on the stove, where my wife was grilling a salmon steak in a black, frying pan. I leaned against the door frame, watching her carefully flip the big, red piece of fish with the spatula. Truly, she was a beautiful woman.

"Smells good."

"Oh." She flinched, looked over at me. "I didn't hear you come in."

"Sorry. Didn't mean to startle you."

She turned to get something from the sink, stopped, stared back at me. "What?"

"What 'what?'"

"What are you looking at me that way for?" She eyed me suspiciously.

"Just looking." From the refrigerator, I grabbed a plastic bottle of Gatorade—cool blue—and unscrewed the top.

"Oh, Margo's housekeeper called. Something about an 'automatic cat box'? She said you'd know what she meant."

"Yeah. I know." I took a big gulp of the cold, pale blue liquid, then remembered—*How soon? How soon?*—and I laughed again.

"What's so funny?"

"'Ees secret.'" I took another sip, then before leaving to shower, leaned against the door frame and asked my wife: "You busy Saturday night?"

She answered with a question: "Why?"

PADDLING-OUT
WITH NEWA

Spring, '08—As a veteran surfer, I'd grown to hate cold water and so didn't surf winters anymore. Each spring when I started surfing again, I liked to leave Pasadena while it was still dark—usually before six a.m.—so I could beat the rush-hour traffic. There's nothing worse than good waves at the beach and being stuck on the freeway, immobilized by a traffic jam. Okay, so cancer's worse. Way-y-y worse. But still, it's a bummer.

I'd lost touch with most of my old surfing buddies or they'd quit riding or passed-away somewhere on my journey through middle-age. Fortunately, my old friend Kurt Gnewuch—who had lost 25 pounds last year—was again willing and able to get back up on his surfboard. He still lived down in Leucadia in North County San Diego. We'd moved there together long ago and had been roommates, sharing houses while I attended SDSU for a couple semesters. We both worked in the construction industry now and there wasn't much work during The Great Recession. So Newa—his nickname since junior-high—articulated a best-case scenario one weekday morning when he called from the shore on his cellphone: "When there's no work, it's my job to surf."

I'd been in the water a few times in full-length wetsuit already that spring and had reacquainted myself with my surfboard—a seven-foot-ten-inch 'tweener (in between a short board and a longboard, sometimes referred to as a fun board in surf-shop lingo). I cruised the 210 east with no problems and transitioned south onto the 605, with slowing only around the Santa Ana Freeway. But by the time I got to the transition to the 405 south, the traffic was already backed up, as usual, even though the sun had barely risen. In between alternative-rock songs on the dashboard radio, morning DJs Kevin & Bean made buffoons of themselves, as usual, and I laughed, as usual, and we inched onto the 405. My cell-phone rang in my pocket; it was Newa's number, so I answered. (It wasn't as if I were driving fast and needed to focus on the road.)

"What's up, Ne?"

"You workin'?"

"Nope. Finished yesterday. Don't start another job till middle of next week. So I'm stuck in four-oh-five traffic with my surfboard strapped to the roof racks. Just another mile and I can exit at Seal Beach Boulevard."

"Stay on the freeway and meet me at Turnarounds. Should be good. Nice swell at Ponto." Ponto was the beach break near his house, close enough that he could see the waves across Pacific Coast Highway from the corner of his block.

But I was only an off-ramp and ten minutes on surface streets away from Sunset Beach, my favorite, local spot (local for me; I surfed there so often spring-through-fall that the real *locals* had long-ago accepted me as one of their own, sociably sharing their waves). "I don't know, Bro. That's another hour-and-a-half in freeway traffic."

"My turn to buy at Beach Break." The Beach Break Café in Oceanside served huge, scrumptious breakfasts, which had become our habit after a morning surf together, usually at Turnarounds, our favorite spot to meet. "I got an hour's work here at the house." He was a carpenter with a makeshift workshop behind his little, back shack of a house. "Call me when you get to San Onofre." It was the nuclear power plant just south of San Clemente. "You got anything better to do with your down-time?"

"Aw, Man." But I really didn't. And my mouth was already watering for those scrambled eggs and hash browns. And I did enjoy surfing with my old buddy. So when we hung up, I poured myself another cup of coffee from the thermos, tore open the pack of Nature Valley granola bars I'd brought from home, and chuckled at Kevin & Bean's shtick, continuing slowly south on the 405 until they were out of range and breaking-up on the coast by San Onofre. I called Kurt to meet me, then tuned-in to the San Diego radio stations, as I drove past Camp Pendleton.

Just south of Carlsbad, Newa's Toyota pick-up was already parked on the dirt lot with a dozen or so other vehicles (there were always more on weekends and once school

15

let out for summer vacation) across PCH from Turnarounds. I parked next to his truck, undressed in my cab, put on my trunks and rash-guard shirt under my full-length wetsuit, then unstrapped my board from the roof racks. I grabbed my pre-packed sports bag—wax, towel, cap, sunscreen, banana, energy gel packets, and sixteen-ounce water bottle—from the back seat and locked the truck cab and shell.

With my board under my other arm, I checked the traffic, then scooted in my sandals across PCH to the top of the cliff, where I looked down on the blue-green ocean under a baby-blue, morning sky. A dozen-plus surfers bobbed like corks on the smooth surface. A four-to-five foot swell rolled in. A black-suited surfer on a small board dropped into the first wave in the set, turned sharply, and scooted across its glassy face, just ahead of the breaking curl, then kicked-out just before it closed-out on the inside. Cool—Newa had guessed right—good waves! And even though the surfers were pretty far away, I picked him out among the scattered group, then climbed hurriedly down the hard, clay face of the shore-side cliff to the sandy, nearly-deserted beach below. (Most families and sunbathers preferred beaches with easier access.)

I put sunscreen on my face and neck, waxed my board, tied its leash around my ankle, and then stepped into the shore break. The water was still chilly. (I hated cold water!) Most of the guys in the water were likewise wearing full-length wetsuits. I waited for a pause between sets, then pushed through an inside breaker, lay on my board, and belly-paddled quickly, trying to get outside before another set crashed in. I barely made it through the impact zone, pushing the nose of my board through the face of a breaking wave—the cold water doused my head and crept into the neck of my wetsuit, making me shiver—then continued to paddle hurriedly towards my buddy Newa. He was wearing a long-sleeved wetsuit with short-legs—a *spring suit* in surf-shop lingo—already acclimated to the springtime water temperature, sitting on his board—a blue, eight-foot 'tweener—waiting for the next set of waves. He smiled when he saw me approaching.

"When's this damn Pacific Ocean going to warm up?" I asked.

"You old guys sure do complain a lot." He was broad-shouldered—like most surfers—with a roundish face—the Caucasian-diluted likeness of his Native American ancestors on his late-father's side—tanned and wrinkled from working and playing in the sun. He'd recently lopped-off his gray-streaked ponytail and sported a more conservative cut.

"It's not *complaining*," I stopped paddling when I got next to him, then sat up on my board. "It's a running commentary."

He laughed. "And that's your job?"

"Apparently."

He reached out a fist and we bumped knuckles. An outside set started to roll in.

"All yours," I said. We were both in good position to catch the first wave, but I figured to wait out this set. Now that I was no longer a kid, I needed to recover my energy for a few minutes after paddling-out.

He turned his board towards shore and started paddling.

"Go get 'em, Ne!" I called after him and watched from behind as the swell lifted his board, then he stood and dropped-in, out of my sight except for his head above the back of the breaking wave, turning left—a natural goofy-footer with his right foot forward—just ahead of the breaking curl, working the wave, then kicking out before the inside. As he paddled back out with a smile on his face, I likewise dropped-in to a fun-sized wave and started ripping. We rode for a couple hours that morning—each rooting the other on like cheerleaders at a football game, neither of us keeping track of time or wipe-outs—before an on-shore wind came up and caused a surface chop, which made the waves crumble over and less ride-able. We each rode a last wave in, exhausted, smiling on the shoreline. It was a good, morning surf and had been worth the drive.

At the back of our trucks in the dirt lot, I poured water from a one-gallon, plastic bottle over my head, then dried off and got dressed in a T-shirt and dry shorts. Kurt did likewise, then we both drove north a few miles to Oceanside, parked on the street, and walked into the Beach Break Café, a small, glass-walled restaurant (next to a likewise-busy laundromat) with surfboards suspended from the ceiling, framed pictures of local surfers ripping the local surf—some signed to the owners Zell and Gary, a fellow surfer—and friendly waitresses in T-shirts, shorts, and tennies. On weekends, the place was always packed with locals and tourists, spilling to umbrella-covered tables outside. But because it was mid-week and brunch-time, we found an empty table inside. A familiar, thirty-something waitress with a blonde ponytail recognized us and brought two cups of coffee without our asking. We exchanged pleasantries, then ordered, and sipped our coffee.

"You hear about that great white killing that triathlete last week?" Kurt asked. "He was swimming right in front of our old house in Solana Beach."

"Yeah, I heard." And I was trying to forget about it! "Damn scary stuff." Neither of us had brought it up earlier because sharks weren't a comfortable subject to broach while sitting on a surfboard with one's legs dangling in the ocean below.

"I was out at Pipes when the lifeguards drove by with their bullhorns: 'Surf at your own risk!' Most everybody paddled-in." He sipped his coffee. "There were only four of us left out in the water for the rest of the day and the waves were *really* good. Next day, too."

"Are you nuts? That damn shark was only a mile away!"

"Dude, when you've got a brain tumor, great white sharks don't mean shit."

We'd known about the tumor at the base of his brain for six months now (a blinding migraine had sent him to the Emergency Room, the cost for which he was still making monthly payments). Its growth was being controlled by drugs—drugs for which Kurt had no medical insurance— that cost him $450 a month out-of-pocket. (Most *worker-bees* in the construction industry didn't carry costly personal policies, especially in this recession.) So his landlord, an old friend and fellow artist like Newa, had told him to forgo the usual $500 rent for the old shack he lived in behind the big, front house. His landlord was presently living in Europe

19

and had rented out the big, front house to a hot, forty-something, surfer lady with long, dark hair and tattoos—one on her deltoid; one on her calf—on whom Kurt had a big crush. But he was too shy with the ladies to let her know. (I pretty much set him up with his first gal pal—a cute, little hippy chick, whom I'd previously dated—in our first house together. But that was another time, another story.) And because of his shyness, he knew she saw him only as a friend.

"Yeah, how you doing with that?" I asked about the tumor not the lady.

"So far, so good. 'Course, they only check me when I can afford another CAT scan. That's like twelve-hundred bucks each time, up front. And it's hard enough paying for the medicine every month. But it's not like it's optional." He pretended to laugh.

All I could do was nod. And even though it was his turn to pay, after we ate, I grabbed the check as soon as our waitress put it on the table. "You can get the tip," I told him but left a couple bucks myself anyway.

As usual, Kurt left a five-dollar bill for our waitress.

Kurt and I surfed together a lot that summer. My mother-in-law owned a condo on the beach at Oceanside (lucky me!) and she let my wife and I use it a few times that year. The water had warmed; Kurt and I wore shorty wetsuits or rash-guard shirts with trunks-only and ripped the waves like kids at an amusement park, sometimes at Turnarounds, sometimes right in front of the condo, anywhere we wanted to paddle-out. Work was still slow, so there was plenty of time for waves. It was a good summer and like-wise fall for surfing. But when the water got cold again as winter approached, I put my surfboard to rest in the corner of our garage at home.

Spring, '09—Kurt and I had started working on a book together that winter. I wrote stories about our adventurous, youthful exploits in Pasadena; he illustrated each in his in-imitably-intertwined, cartoon-like fashion. I'd send him a scene, describe what I envisioned, then he'd e-mail back his sketches. Most of my critiquing involved his habit of put-ting thumbs or toes in the wrong direction due to his dys-lexia. We laughed about it. It wasn't a problem as long as I caught each misdirected digit before he inked in the pencil sketches. We surfed together a few times that spring. But he was getting weaker, losing more weight, and by the end of June, couldn't risk paddling-out any more. He began going back for more tests—costly tests. (I'd been riding him for months to sign up for Medi-Cal, which he'd finally done.) My wife and I were staying at the condo for a few days, so I drove down to Leucadia and picked him up (he didn't feel like driving). We had breakfast as usual at the Beach Break Café. (He didn't eat much, taking most of his omelet and hash browns in a to-go container for later at home.) My turn to buy and he left his usual five-dollar tip.

I drove him to the condo, where we sat under the *palapa* on the private beach above the public beach and sipped cool, iced drinks like millionaires on vacation. He and my wife talked. She was a Special Ed teacher. He opened up— something he rarely did with a woman—explaining to her about his own problems in elementary school:

"They didn't call it dyslexia back then—they just called me dumb."

They talked for the better part of an hour. I didn't butt in. I just watched the waves from behind my Ray-Bans. It was a little windy; the ocean was choppy; the waves weren't good for surfing. But it was hot on the beach. So when Kurt and my wife were done talking, I suggested: "Let's go get wet."

"You two go," my wife advised.

So Kurt and I stepped down the steps from our private beach—he holding the handrail—to the public beach below and strolled slowly across the hot sand to the cool shoreline, where we stepped into the shore break. A wave splashed over our knees; he wobbled and pretended to laugh.

"Don't let me drown, Bro."

I stood next to him. "I won't."

He pretended to laugh again. "Might not be a bad way to go."

"Might not." Another small wave washed over our knees. "But not today."

He smiled. "No, not today."

The tattooed surfer lady in the front house threw a party for Kurt over the weekend. All his friends from North County showed up. Kurt called me the next day, said it had been a really good party, even though he couldn't eat much—any—of the food they had prepared. The following Monday, he went to see the oncologist who had ordered the tests. On his way home from the doctor's office that afternoon, he called me from his truck on the freeway:

"Goddamn cancer metastasized. Got a tumor the size of a softball attached to my liver. And they can't operate for some damn reason! Two weeks, Man!" There was a pause, then he repeated, more quietly: "Two weeks—then I'm dead."

"Ah, shit, Ne. Wh-what about chemo?"

"Yeah, the doctor's submitting the paperwork to Medi-Cal. But it takes a week or two for it to go through and get approval. And he said it probably wouldn't do any good anyway." His voice dropped off, barely audible: "It's progressed too far."

I took off work the next day, stopped by another old friend's house, then drove down south. I got off the freeway in Oceanside, got some scrumptious crumb cake to-go at the Beach Break Café (they were moving to a new and larger location next year), then drove down to Kurt's. He was sitting alone in the overgrown back yard with his black cat nearby.

"What's happenin', you ol' hippie surfer."

He looked over from his garden chair and tried to smile. But he was gaunt and there was no life in his thinning, deeply-wrinkled face. A half-dozen, empty Ensure bottles sat motionless, collecting dust on the wooden, spool table between us. I pushed them aside and put the to-go bag on the table.

"Have you been eating?"

"Can't. No appetite. And sometimes I throw up when I try." He paused before adding: "It's really getting to me, Bro."

I reached into my pocket and pulled out a small, green plastic container with a prescription label—filled with buds—and put it on the table between us. "You have a pipe?"

He looked over, saw the container, and laughed a little. "I tried that at the party. Didn't help. Just made me paranoid."

"This is medical-grade marijuana, not that commercial, Mexican weed they smuggle over the border down here. Friend of mine has a card."

He nodded, unconvinced. "I don't have a pipe or papers." We hadn't smoked pot together since our dippy-hippy days in the century past. "There's a lighter on the stove inside."

So I made a pipe from one of the empty Ensure bottles and a piece of aluminum foil (necessity—the mother of invention), put in a bud, each took a hit and held it. As I exhaled, I could feel my eyelids lower immediately. I smiled and handed him the pipe again, lit the lighter. He leaned in and took another hit, exhaled, smiled, too. We each took a few more hits, coughed, handing the pipe and lighter back and forth, then both just sat there, spaced-out, staring at his cat, sneaking through the underbrush after a lizard in the overgrown garden, both of us silently mesmerized by the hunt. But the skink slithered away before the cat could pounce. The cat looked up at Kurt, as if to explain.

"He likes to leave their carcasses on my doorstep."

"Yeah, I had an ex-girlfriend like that once." It didn't make any sense, but we both cracked-up laughing anyway. We exchanged a few *remember-that-time* stories, laughing some more at our old antics together. He'd finished the art-work for nine of the stories in our book before running out of energy, life. (I later got each story published—a website here, a literary journal there—featuring Newa's animated illustrations.)

I took the to-go bag inside, heated up the crumb cakes in their individual, cardboard containers in the micro-wave along with the plastic container of icing, then went back out-side. I placed the crumb cakes on the wooden, spool table between us, then handed him a plastic fork.

"Hmm," he said, contemplating—to eat or not to eat?

I took the container of icing and poured half over the top of his treat, then over mine. They were big, fat pieces. I picked up my plastic fork.

"On three," I directed, then skipped *one* and *two*: "Three." And dug into the corner of my icing-laden crumb cake, taking it slowly into my mouth, emphasizing: "Mm-m-m."

He smiled and did likewise.

Later, I left him the container of medicine for his chemo treatments. "You'll probably need it."

But Kurt never made it to his chemo treatments and wasn't around for the opening of the new-and-improved Beach Break Café. Because thirteen days after his oncolo-gist's two-week prognosis—the day before he was to start chemotherapy—he passed-out in his kitchen, where the tat-tooed surfer lady from the front house later found him on the floor. She called the paramedics, but it was too late. At the hospital, they put him on life-support, until his friends and family could pay our last respects. Worst drive to North County I ever made. I tried to prepare myself. His Mom, whom I hadn't seen since Kurt and I were in high school, the tattooed surfer lady, and some other family members were in the hospital room, too, when I got there. But when I saw him lying motionless in that hospital bed with that respirator shoved down his throat—artificially pumping oxygen into his lungs, keeping his heart beating—I lost it, Bro.

A month later, I gave his eulogy on the beach near his house at Ponto. Kurt's mom had T-shirts made for all of us with his working-class mantra on front, *"When there's no work, it's my job to surf."* and a smiling, young Kurt with a Christmas-present surfboard on back. She handed out *leas*, too, which we all wore around our necks. I hadn't written anything down beforehand. I figured it'd come to me. I figured that's the way Ne would've wanted it. I remembered starting: "I first met Kurt Gnewuch when I was ten years old. He was nine..." But it was pretty much a blur after that. Somehow, I made it through without blubbering. Just barely. (My thigh was later-bruised from pinching it each time I started to ball-up.) I kept my sunglasses on—just in case. When I was done, Kurt's mom gave me a back-sling with his ashes inside. We all grabbed our surfboards, posed on the beach for a final picture, then hit the surf. The water was warm but the waves were consistent, and so I struggled to paddle-out with Newa's ashes around my neck in the back-sling. And unfortunately, I'd forgotten to take off my sunglasses. So I bid farewell to both my Ray-Bans and my last, best surfing buddy that day. Once we paddled-out past the breakers, we all formed a circle on our surfboards. Each told a personal story about our friend Kurt, then I paddled to the center and opened the back-sling, spreading his ashes on the ocean. Each of us tossed our *leas* in the center, too. As funerals go, Newa's *paddle-out* was a damn good one.

At the wake afterwards, I got a drink, excused myself from my wife ("I'll be right back."), then sidled up next to the tattooed surfer lady and told her in private:

"You know—Kurt had a big crush on you."

"Really?" She smiled. Her dark eyes stared back into mine.

"Yeah. I figured you should know."

"Yeah." We clinked our plastic, cocktail glasses together, toasting Kurt. "Thanks," she said.

On his last conscious day, Kurt and I had been talking on our cellphones when he said: "If I don't make it through this, Bro—write my story."

"Damn, Ne, that's an awful lot of pressure," I admitted, but told him anyway: "I already have the title—'Paddling-Out with Newa.'"

He was quiet for a moment, then admitted: "I like it."

"Yeah. I figured you would."

MARK BARKAWITZ

WAVING GOODBYE

Kurt Gnewuch aka the artist Newa—gentle soul, hard-
working carpenter, good friend, and generous tipper.
(The waitresses will miss him, too.)
Veteran goofy-foot surfer, who lived by his simple mantra:
"When there's no work, it's my job to surf."
9/30/'51 — 8/14/'09
Last Paddle-Out — 9/12/'09

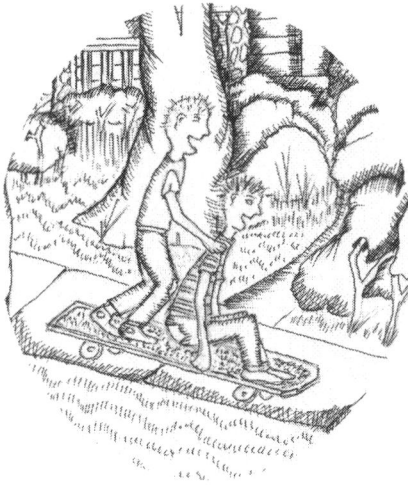

MARK BARKAWITZ

THE CHEMO LOUNGE

Fall, '10—And then it was my turn to fight for my life. . .

My back had broken from the incurable blood and bone cancer that battered my entire body. So I wasn't able to steer my truck to my chemotherapy treatments without a great deal of pain—twice a week for two weeks, then a week off to let my body recover from the powerful drugs. As such, my mother-in-law volunteered to drive me. Marian was a classy-looking, older woman who mostly dressed in black and gold with diamonds in gold jewelry, make-up, and a platinum-streaked coif. She drove a gold Cadillac. Her husband Bob had passed-away a few years prior from pancreatic cancer, about which little could be done. I think driving me empowered her—at least this time she could do something—to help fight the culprit that had taken her husband of 49 years. So the medical staff and nurses at my oncologist Dr. Hu's office saw the two of us together regularly when I came in for my treatments.

Most of the nurses and office staff were of Asian or Filipino descent. Except for Carmen the receptionist, always seated at the computer behind the counter, smiling as she took co-pays and checked for insurance when we entered, then assigning each patient to our next office visit before we exited.

The routine was much the same each time. After my name was called, Karen—in nurse's scrubs—checked my weight and blood pressure at one end of the hallway. She would then lead me to an examination room if I were to see Dr. Hu or—if for treatment only—to The Chemo Lounge, as I referred to it: a large, blue-walled room filled with a half-dozen recliners with IV stands next to each, privacy curtains hanging from the ceiling, and a couple of strategically-placed, flat-screen TVs. Each recliner was usually filled with a patient who was there for treatment, which typically lasted for hours. (Mine took from an hour-to-2½ hours to complete, depending on what they were putting into me that day.) I always came prepared with the Sports section of the newspaper, a *TIME* magazine, munchies—granola bars or a peanut butter and jelly sandwich my wife had made for me—and a box juice. I usually read. Sometimes, I watched TV. Sometimes, I put on my ear-buds, closed my eyes, and listened to music on my iPod. Occasionally, I had a conversation with the patient in the next recliner. But most of us felt lousy from our illnesses and/or the treatments, so there wasn't a lot of socialization. We were more like a barroom full of solitary drunks, each wallowing separately with our IV cocktails. Even so, I was the gabby type; it helped pass the time. So I'd welcome the newbies if they sat nearby—you could tell by the looks on their faces if it was their first intravenous treatment—helping them feel more comfortable—*You're not alone*—in this odd setting. And I spoke regularly with the nurses. Got to know each over time, as they stuck the intravenous needle into the vein in the crook of my arm. ("No pain, no pain, no pain," was a mantra I repeated quickly whenever I got stuck, which was an awful lot for a guy like me, who used to hate needles but now relied on them for my very existence.) The IV tube led to a bag of Velcade or Doxil to kill my cancer cells or Zometa to strengthen my greatly weakened bones. Each treatment was specialized to each patient. Dr. Hu read the numbers from our blood-work and devised each formula according to our specific cancer—multiple myeloma, in my case—and needs. He had a reputation for keeping a lot of people alive for a long time, so I felt lucky indeed to have been referred to him by my primary-care physician in our HMO.

I had improved greatly over the past few months from near-dead and propped-up on a walker to ambling cautiously without one. Dr. Hu's head nurse Amy had predicted as much after my first cycle. ("Next time you come here, you won't need that walker.") And she'd been right, for which I hugged her. We always hugged now—I felt an affinity for her and most of the staff, each doing their parts to help keep me alive—when we passed in the hallway or if she stopped by my examination room while Dr. Hu was still with another patient.

At the start of each new cycle, Dr. Hu—tall, calm, with graying hair and metal-rimmed glasses—read my latest blood-work chart on the computer and reported a higher percentage of cancer had been eradicated by my previous cycle of treatment. So my motto soon became: chemo in; cancer out! Sure, I felt lousy—really lousy—but it was working! Of course, I still had the broken back—for which I would receive surgery only if I survived the cancer—so even though I was getting stronger, I was still in a lot of pain and still needed a ride twice a week to my treatments, which lasted for six months.

I only saw Jerome—who mixed the chemo drugs in Dr. Hu's formulas—behind a paper breather-mask, rubber gloves, and full, safety apron, like some mad scientist who held our lives in his capable hands. He'd sometimes seek me out in the Chemo Lounge between mixing batches to talk for a minute or two. He was Filipino with Catholic roots and had confessed to me that he offered up each batch to the heavens for the Lord's blessing. I thanked him for his earnestness and told him:

"It's working."

I couldn't see his mouth behind the mask, but the glint in his eyes told me he smiled.

Marian had to go out of town for a week, so my wife took a sick-day at work—which she'd lose if she didn't use it—and drove me to my chemo appointment. Suzanna was nearly ten years younger than I and looked even more so now that I was beat-up and bent-over from the cancer, broken back, and chemo. She worked-out regularly—a long, lean, natural blonde, who barely/rarely wore make-up, unlike her mother. Carmen looked up and smiled when we walked in together and glanced over a few times as we waited in the waiting room. Karen likewise gave us a double-take when she called my name. At the time, I didn't think anything of it.

For the last treatment in that cycle, my daughter Carly—between classes at Pasadena City College—drove me. A look-a-like, flashback version of my wife but wearing make-up (it skipped a generation) with a pink streak dyed into her shoulder-length hair, she sat with me in the waiting room, engrossed in her iPhone screen. Once again, Carmen glanced over, smiling to herself.

After my week off, I'd just start to feel better as the effects of the chemo started to wear off when it was time again to start another cycle. I reminded myself: chemo in; cancer out! Marian was back in town and drove me. Carmen was her usual smiling self. Karen, too.

After another encouraging report from Dr. Hu, I sat in an empty recliner in the Chemo Lounge, which was mostly empty that morning because I had an early appointment. It would fill-up soon. When one of the nurses came over with my bag of chemo, we exchanged our usual greetings. I asked about her family. She said all was fine. But then she asked me: "Can I ask you a question?"

"Sure." I started my mantra as she stuck the IV needle into my vein: "No pain, no pain no pain."

"Some of us were wondering." She taped the IV needle to the crook of my arm, then spoke more intimately: "Which one of the ladies is your wife?"

I couldn't help laughing. "Marian's my mother-in-law," I explained, pointing towards the waiting room. "I can't drive because of my back. And my wife works. She was in here a couple weeks ago. Tall, blonde, attractive."

"Oh, yes, I remember. All attractive. The youngest?"

"Daughter."

She nodded. "Of course."

As Marian and I walked out to the upper-level parking lot, I shared with her: "The nurses and office staff thought I was your boy-toy."

"What?" She stopped in her tracks, staring over at me behind her designer sunglasses.

I nodded. "Yep. Then when Suzanna and Carly showed up, they weren't sure which of you was my wife. Funny, huh?"

"Boy, you're not kidding."

We both laughed. It felt good to laugh. Before the chemo made me sick again in the next few days. But what the heck—chemo in; cancer out—The Chemo Lounge was working!

MARATHON MAN

I got my stem cell transplant on June 6, 2011 at City of Hope Hospital. As Helena the nurse hung the IV bag with my reconditioned stem cells—autologous; self-donated—she said to me:

"Congratulations, today is your new birthday." She spoke behind a paper breather-mask and wore blue, nitrile gloves for my protection. "Happy birthday, Marathon Man."

"Thanks, Helena."

The staff in the hospital had already taken to calling me Marathon Man because I usually wore one of my L.A. Marathon T-shirts on my daily walk around the corridors of our wing. I likewise had to wear nitrile gloves and a paper breather-mask when I left my environmentally-controlled room, so my face was partially-obscured to the nurses and doctors at their stations and other patients in their rooms with their doors and curtains sometimes opened like neighbors. Thus my T-shirt—with its stickman personification of runners under a palm tree—was my most prominent feature; that and my full head of hair, the roots of which had somehow held snugly—unlike most of the other male patients in this wing—throughout my cancer treatments thus far. The trek around our wing was 1/8th of a mile—I tried to do a-mile-a-day—so most saw me repeatedly on my laps, often giving me the thumbs-up signal, sometimes cheering me on: "Go, Marathon Man!"

It was a hopeful day for me all right but far from *happy*. 95% of the cancer in my system had been obliterated by six months of chemo, two massive doses of which they'd IVed into me two days prior. And I still had a broken back from the blood and bone cancer—multiple myeloma—that had spawned in and deteriorated my marrow, so I was in a lot of pain. But there was hope now that I could actually beat this thing. I decided to give myself a birthday present and took the day off from my walk. I threw-up instead.

When I awoke the morning after my new birthday, my pillowcase was covered with hair. Damn. I didn't know if it was the result of the double-dose of chemo—the strongest my system had yet endured—or the stem cell transplant. Didn't matter. I brushed it carefully in the mirror but my hair collected in the bristles. And in the shower drain. And on my bath towel.

I held out a couple more days, then asked Helena the nurse to shave my head like the others. It looked okay in the mirror, but my naked noggin was freezing cold! The knitted cap they'd supplied me made my scalp and forehead itch. So I took a T-shirt and stuck the neck hole over my head down to my ears, wearing it like a pharaoh's headdress until my bald head acclimated itself to the coolness of the room's controlled climate. Who knew?

To harvest my stem cells and because the entire transplant process required so much intravenous work, my new oncologist Dr. Htut (pronounced "Tut" like the long-ago Egyptian king) at City of Hope had prescribed a Hickman catheter for my treatment. As such, I'd had tubes surgically-implanted just below my neck, attached to my subclavian vein and some artery down in my chest. Sort of like a bolo tie with an *insie* and an *outsie* hose. I hated it at first—having to clean it daily so the incision wouldn't get infected, the way it hung out of my chest like a symbol of my infirmity— but it sure was useful in here. During my entire incarceration (that's what it felt like), I never got stuck with a single needle! The nurses just hung an IV bag with whatever Dr. Htut wanted to put inside of me and screwed it into my Hickman catheter. *Voila!* So unlike most of the other patients who likewise walked the halls, I was one of the few who didn't have to drag along my IV bag (or bags) on a stainless-steel, *me-and-my-shadow* IV stand on wheels. The nurses just unscrewed me each day around noon for my daily walks—the best part of my days. So even with my broken back, I usually lapped the other patients. *Go, Marathon Man! Go!*

Because my immune system was compromised, I was scheduled to spend three weeks in isolation like all other autologous transplant patients (six weeks if it's somebody else's donor cells, so I tried not to complain). Oh sure, I could have visitors. But they had to wear masks and gloves and the whole rigmarole and to be truthful, I felt lousy and really didn't like entertaining people, making conversation (highly unusual for yours truly). So except on weekends, I mostly phoned my wife and kids and texted my friends.

There's not a lot to do when you're isolated in an isolation unit. I kept telling myself: *Three weeks is over in three weeks.* I tried not to look at the calendar on the wall that first week. But the days were interminably long. I crossed off each with a black "X." I refused to watch TV before four o'clock, which gave me something to look forward to each afternoon, unless it was the weekend and there was an early game on. Each morning, I tried to bribe the food service guy or the custodian with a five-dollar bill to get me the *L.A. Times* from the newsstand downstairs. Because I had *chemo-brain*—short term memory loss from chemotherapy—I got to read the Sports section twice!

I couldn't keep food down, so they fed me intravenously. But I knew they wouldn't cut me loose until I could eat solid food again, so I tried daily and threw-up daily. Because they'd replaced my toothbrush with a mini-sponge on a cardboard stick—minimizing the risk of my gums bleeding and infecting—I just couldn't get a fresh feeling inside my mouth, even after gargling. I longed for my toothbrush!

There's a lot of discomfort involved with long-distance running. Successful runners learned to disregard the brain's efforts to halt the body's nonstop locomotion with a mind-over-matter *modus operandi*—it doesn't matter if it hurts, I'm running! You learned to push through pain. And once the endorphins started flowing, it was almost like a self-induced state of perpetual motion. Admittedly, it was impossible to get those same endorphins secreting on my strolls around the hospital halls, but I put on my iPod ear-buds and forged through my laps anyway. The T-shirts with the racing stickmen (whom I physically-resembled now) were a reminder of the most difficult physical act I had previously achieved—six months of intense training, leading to a 3:44:42 race time over the 26.2 mile course. But admittedly, recovering from incurable cancer and a broken back made running the marathon feel like child's play.

I was weak as a newborn, all right, but started doing arm curls while in bed with a dumbbell bar—just the bar; no weights attached; my weakened muscles and unstable spine couldn't handle more—that I'd brought in my luggage from home. Eight days after my stem cell transplant, I was able to eat solid food again and keep it down. I worked back up to my mile-a-day walks. Seventeen days after I'd been admitted, Dr. Htut agreed to my early release. It was shortest stint for an autologous stem cell transplant that anyone on staff could remember. *Go, Marathon Man! Go home!* To my wife and my kids and my toothbrush! *Voila!*

Because it had served its purpose, the Hickman catheter was removed from my chest in an out-patient procedure a week later. *Adios, Amigo!* And having two birthdays a year now sounded pretty cool. I was actually looking forward to getting my back fused next (no pain—no gain). Who knew:

Maybe the doctors and nurses at City of Hope could put me back together again? So far—so good! I figured to check with Dr. Htut about the record for multiple myeloma survival. Because Marathon Man intended to break that, too!

A PRETTY GOOD DEAL

Helena the nurse shaved my head today. I'd been contemplating it ever since my lock-down in here. Only took about half-an-hour. Kept the short beard (for now).

Staring in the mirror, I appear a cross between Bruce Willis and a retired, cage fighter. Didn't take but a few moments for me to get accustomed to my new look. (I'm sure it's more traumatic for the ladies.)

I haven't been out of my environmentally-controlled room yet. Walking the halls in my breather mask and blue, nitrile gloves, I'm pretty sure I'll get a few second looks. But most of the men in here have their domes likewise fashioned; one gets tired of leaving all that hair on the pillowcase. So when I leave City of Hope next week, it'll be hair-free and cancer-free.

All-in-all, a pretty good deal.

MARK BARKAWITZ

SICK AS a DOG

Back when I was *really* sick—down to 122 lbs. with a broken back, propped on a four-wheeled walker with hand brakes—my dogs still wanted to walk. And I wanted to walk, too. Heck, I wasn't dead. Not yet anyway. So one day, I got the bright idea of tying Summa—the larger but more controllable of my two golden retrievers—with her leash to the front of my walker. I put on the ear-buds of my iPod, sucked down some energy gel, and we strolled slowly onto the sidewalk. When she pulled too fast, I partially-applied both hand brakes and ordered:

"Slow down, Summa."

We made it to the corner without any hitches. I could only imagine what my neighbors must've thought. I'd been a distance runner most of my life. Lifted weights in my garage. Surfed every summer, too. Until one day while training for a half-marathon, a vertebra in my lower back suddenly broke. Hurt like hell! My orthopedist diagnosed it the result of a birth defect in my spine. *Birth defect? At my age?* That was ridiculous, and I told him so. Our relationship and my health spiraled downward. Seven doctors and nine months later—keeled-over with an all-over-body-pain in my primary-care physician's office—Dr. Gomez explained:

"You have multiple myeloma, Mark."

I lifted my head. "Is that a gum disease or cancer?" I'm kind of a smart ass. Sometimes. But I really didn't know.

"It's cancer of the blood and bone marrow. I'm sorry."

I must've sighed deeply, because all the air left my being. As a lifelong athlete, I knew my body well, and it had been telling me for a long time that something—not only my wrecked spine—was wrong. But *this* was my worst fear. "Am I going to die?"

"Fifty/fifty." Then he quickly recalculated: "With you— make it sixty/forty. Better than Vegas odds." He'd been my doctor for years and knew me pretty well.

I pretended to laugh.

"The cancer has shut down your kidneys. Our primary concern right now is to get them functioning again. Otherwise, you're going to be dead in two days." He put his hand on my shoulder. "Better make plans—just in case."

45 minutes later, I sat in a recliner at Urgent-Care with an IV needle in the large, bluish vein in the crook of my arm, contemplating my mortality.

We turned south at the corner. It was mid-day midweek, so there wasn't much traffic. Another golden named *Finicce* (Italian for Phoenix, the mythological bird reborn from ashes) was sometimes loose on his front lawn while his owner Justin read the newspaper on their porch. Summa didn't like other big dogs. And sensing my weakened condition, she'd become aggressively defensive of me. But fortunately, Finicce wasn't outside today. I was relieved. My most immediate concern wasn't the cancer coursing through my veins but a loose dog or cat or Summa's favorite—squirrels, which populated the neighborhood trees. Chasing was no longer within my physical ability. Slow was my only speed. I had a limp now, too—left leg—from the cancer in my hip. X-rays revealed it had spread to every bone in my body—even my freakin' skull!

Yep, I was *sick as a dog*, all right. Funny expression. Dogs aren't necessarily sick at all. Probably Shakespearean in origin. From a time when God's creatures were believed to exist on different levels: the angels above, the beasts below. So when a man became out of sorts—afflicted with melancholy—his level lowered to that of a dog. I think. But it's a long time since college. And I had chemo-brain now—short-term memory loss from chemotherapy—which was only temporary. But then—so was I.

At the southeast corner, we made another right turn onto Orange Grove Boulevard. It was warm for early December. But Southern California was often like that. So I'd put on sunscreen, a baseball cap, and sunglasses with my T-shirt and nylon track pants. My clothes hung loosely on me now like a hanger. A few cars whizzed past. I felt oddly out of place and time, like an old jockey harnessed behind his horse in a seat-less sulky. I tried to pick up the pace. But that didn't last long. The cancer—and chemo—sucked my energy. Heck, I just wanted to make it around the damn block! I hit the brakes again slightly.

"Slow down, Summa."

Up ahead, a large Rottweiler patrolled his property behind a wrought iron fence and electronically-controlled
gates. As we approached, Summa pulled harder—she knew
where he lived, too.

"Whoa, whoa, whoa," I said above a whisper, braking. I
didn't want my voice alerting the Rottie either. But Summa
continued to pull, her chest heaving, her breathing rasped by
the linked-chain collar pulled tighter around her neck. I continued braking, but the back wheels only slid. The big-
headed Rottie lay in wait. Summa jerked us forward until
both dogs were at each other face-to-face with the wrought
iron's mesh between them, making loud, vicious noises but
unable to do each other any harm.

"Summa! Stop!" I pulled back on the walker. "Stop-p-
p!"

She continued to snarl her teeth but backed off. The Rottie raced behind the fence to the western gate and stood
panting, waiting for our next encounter. I tried to steer
closer to the parkway grass, but at nearly-ninety pounds and
with four-footed drive, Summa's strength out-matched
mine. They went at it again with the gate between them until I convinced Summa to pass. The honey-colored fur on her
back stood-up straight like a warning—*DON'T MESS WITH
ME!* That Rottie would've kicked her butt. But she remained fearless, defiant. I laughed and wished I had her
courage to likewise face my foe.

There were no more dogs on this side of the block. I re-
membered my iPod in my pocket and turned it on. The
Wallflowers sang of driving home *"with o-one headlight."*
Partially-impaired. Physically and metaphorically. The ob-

jective correlative—something which stands by itself while mutually representing something else in the story. But my walker had *no-o headlights* at all. So where in hell did that leave me?

We turned north—right turn number three—at the corner. The purplish-green San Gabriel Mountains stood serrated below the intensely blue sky. We were more than halfway. Thank God. My legs, which had carried me over 10,000 miles in my distance-running past, were already tired. The bone pain from the cancer was sometimes mind-blowing. But today—so far—it was bearable. (The two Vicodin I'd popped earlier helped greatly.) I steered us down a driveway because a pit bull lived up at the corner. But as I strained to look over my shoulder—twisting was painful with my unstable spine—a work truck with ladders atop sped closely past in the street. I squeezed the brakes hard, "Whoa!" to stop Summa in front of me. In my ear-buds, the late Amy Winehouse mellifluously refused to *"go to rehab"* (her fatal mistake), so I hadn't heard the truck. I took a deep breath and sighed. Summa looked back.

"My bad."

But she didn't seem to mind my tunnel-vision. Cancer had a way of doing that to a guy—narrowing one's vision. Or to a gal. It certainly wasn't sexist. Or racist. Or even classist. No, cancer was an equal-opportunity killer. I looked both ways and crossed to the other sidewalk. My hip ached. Just make it to flat ground at the corner.

We did, eventually, and negotiated a wide, right-turn-number-four out into the street onto our side of the block. From the corner house, the pit bull barked at us. Summa and I looked over, but he was hidden behind the cinder block wall. Sometimes, the scariest things of all were unseen.

I steered us up a driveway onto the sidewalk. Only a half-block left. Cool. I was going to make it. A pleasant, little ditty—"Birdhouse in Your Soul"—came on. I took out my iPod to turn up the volume and so didn't see the squirrel ahead on the parkway grass. But Summa did. And because I had the iPod in one hand, I only held the walker with the other, which suddenly yanked me forward, face-first onto the sidewalk—"Umph!"—and out of my grasp. Once again, all the air collapsed from my being. When I looked up, Summa with my four-wheeled walker bouncing behind was in hot pursuit of the squirrel, who barely beat her to the base of a jacaranda, the trunk of which it scaled as if shot from a canon. Summa leapt teeth-first—she had tasted squirrel before—just missing its bushy tail. Then she jumped up against the tree as if on tiptoes, staring up, the leashed-walker lying idly behind on its side—one wheel still spinning.

Looking back on that episode in my recovery, I'd be hard-pressed to call it a wholly-successful leap forward in physical therapy. (Face-forward maybe?) But after six months of chemotherapy, a stem cell transplant at our good neighbors the City of Hope, and neurosurgery to implant titanium rods in my spine, Summa and I—reborn like the Phoenix from ashes—were up to three-miles-a-day when we walked. Without the walker. Or the limp. Or the cancer. I was a light-welterweight again. Resumed bench-pressing (carefully) in my garage. I walked my other dog again now, too, even though she was wildly exuberant, even at the end of a leash. And now that yours truly was no longer *sick as a dog*, I was pretty damn exuberant, too!

MARK BARKAWITZ

ELECTRIFIED!

"Not tonight," his wife said in the dark. "I just got my period."

Mike rolled away from her in their bed. In the old days, Hannah would always warn him: "We'd better do it tonight because I'm about to get my period." Not anymore. Now, it was an extended excuse. He tried to understand. It wasn't as if they were young lovers anymore. Their twentieth wedding anniversary was next month. Their sex life had been good for a long time. But with two teenage kids in the house, his opportunities to *get lucky*, as she put it, were limited. He closed his eyes in the dark and tried not to think about it.

Sunday morning, he got up early and went for a five-mile run down to Old Town and back. Clouds had backed up over the nearby San Gabriel Mountains and obscured the sun. Good running weather. But his legs felt heavy and his neoprene-wrapped ankle ached with a nagging injury that had kept him off the streets for long periods of rehab over the last year-and-a-half. But he wasn't happy if he wasn't running, so he pushed himself through the pain. He was about three miles into his run on Colorado Boulevard when from behind he was suddenly passed by a dark, dangling ponytail attached to a lithe, lean female runner in a yellow top and red shorts. She didn't look back. Hmm. He picked up his pace. Hers remained steady. He was able to stay with her—a half-dozen steps behind—for the next couple blocks. But eventually, he got winded and his quads fatigued. The traffic light a half-block ahead was green but blinked: "DON'T WALK." She kicked it up another notch and ran through the yellow light at the corner. A few more steps behind, he stopped for the red light, panting, bent-over, hands propped on his knees. She didn't bother to look back.

He stopped for water at Jefferson Park. Splashed his face. Down the back of his neck. Leaned on the rock and concrete fountain before starting the final mile of his run. She had kicked his butt as if he were an old man. A couple of young, Latino guys kicked a soccer ball around on the park grass. He took another drink. No way she runs by me like that two years ago. Damn ankle. No damn way.

That afternoon, he rode the Metro-Rail Gold Line from Pasadena to the Red Line train in Hollywood and got off with his backpack at Children's Hospital in Los Angeles to visit a sick friend. "CD" was a seventh-grader on the school track team that he coached. (He had nicknames for most of his student-athletes.) She ran the mile, the longest of the events for middle-schoolers. But two weeks ago at their Saturday practice, she was winded from running a warm-up lap on the track with the rest of the team and her skin color had a yellowish tinge. He sat her out for the rest of practice. Her father took her to the doctor the following Monday. She was diagnosed with leukemia. It had shocked the whole team. They voted her team captain and had a cap made for her that was embroidered: "CD - Team Captain." One of the parents solicited donations to help the family. It being a parochial school, there was a lot of praying and candle-lighting in the church, too. But there was only so much you could do.

Even though he had wrapped his ankle in ice after his morning run, it was beginning to throb again on the elevator ride up to CD's floor. He got off on a floor with brightly-decorated walls painted with clowns, balloons, and smiling animals. The decorators had endeavored to make it a cheery place, but everywhere he looked there were sick kids in hospital beds, some with hair, some with little, some without any. A tall administrator led an older gentleman wearing an ascot and crested blazer down the hallway past him. Mike overheard her explain: "In the old days, this was the place where children came to die." Mike wanted to hear what it was now, but they continued to walk away from him.

He found CD's room. She was sitting in bed, looking bored but her skin was no longer yellow, thanks to the blood transfusion which had corrected her white cell count. She had an IV in her arm. Her mother Elena—mid-thirties, Latina, with a girlish figure—sat in a chair at the foot of the bed. Her father John—a slightly-built, dark-haired man, who had been a distance runner himself in high school— stood staring out the window.

"Hi, CD." They all turned, as if looking for Hope to enter the room, but it was only him. The family smiled the same, weary half-smiles.

"Hi, Coach," CD said.

He wanted to bump knuckles with her—their usual track team greeting—but wasn't sure if he should touch her. A lot of the kids in the hospital wore paper breather-masks to ward off infection and he noticed one on the nightstand near her bed. So he nodded to her and shook her father's hand instead ("Thanks for coming, Mike.") and hugged her mother. ("Good to see you, Coach Mike.") He tried to be upbeat but it seemed forced even to himself. Then he re-membered the cap in the backpack.

"Here." He handed it to CD. "We voted you team cap-tain. Unanimously."

She forced another smile. CD liked being the center of attention—a young, drama queen—but this wasn't a part she wanted to play. She pulled the cap on over her mane of thick, black hair, which she would probably lose in the com-ing months from the chemo. He told CD about their recent track meet and her teammates' exploits and antics and how he expected her to be back running for the team next year, but it was as if he could hear himself talking, saying one thing while wanting to shout out loud how damn unfair this was to all these little kids to be this damn sick! Instead, he tried to be cheery. *Cheery.* He hugged her mom goodbye, then reached over to squeeze CD's big toe, which was under

the covers (a common safe-practice he'd previously ob-
served in children's wards). She nodded back but didn't
smile. Her father walked him out. They spoke quietly in the
hallway.

"The doctor said she's only had it for a few weeks."
John's eyes were bloodshot, sagging with exhaustion. "It's
good they found it early."

He nodded back. "Yeah."

"We just got the tests back. It's a treatable strain. Thank
God." John sighed, as if all the air had been let out of his
body.

Mike nodded again.

"Eighty percent survival rate."

"That's good."

It was John's turn to nod. "She goes on chemo in the
next week or so. Every three weeks for nine months." He
struggled to make it to the next sentence. "My wife quit her
job to stay with her. I haven't been to work either since she
was diagnosed." He seemed as if he wanted to say more.

Mike hugged CD's father. He didn't know what else to
do.

Monday morning, Mike drove his kids to school. On the
way, his daughter Alice, a fourteen-year-old image of her
mother, complained from the passenger seat of the truck's
quad-cab: "We have to get a new computer. That thing is so
slow now. It's taking me forever to do my term paper."

"We bought that computer three years ago," Mike
pointed out, while maneuvering through the rush-hour traffic. "It can't be worn-out already."

"It's a piece of crap," his eighteen-year-old son Peter chimed in from the back seat. He had a new laptop, a gift for last spring's high school graduation.

"I'll take a look at it," Mike said.

"You?" his son scoffed, already inches taller than his father. "What are you gonna do?"

In the front seat, Alice agreed by laughing with her brother. Pete patted him on the shoulder. "That's a good one, Pops."

Admittedly, Mike's computer skills were limited. But he was used to fixing things himself—one way or another. He dropped Alice off at her private high school and Pete at Pasadena City College, then drove to Marten's Restaurant to finish some minor repair work in their kitchen. (He didn't charge for coaching kids, but he surely did for fixing-up greasy, commercial kitchens.) The restaurant was closed for the week for repairs and remodeling, most of which he had completed. But when he arrived, the old dishwasher was still leaking—even though the repairman had been out over the weekend—and had soaked the lower part of a wall he still had to paint. Bill the owner—eyes tired from too much work and stress but in good physical shape from riding his mountain bike regularly—explained the repairmen were due back that morning.

"Could you let them in? I have to get out of here. This is *supposed* to be my vacation."

Mike said sure and then unloaded equipment from his truck. His ankle was already starting to ache, so he popped the last, two aspirins from the first-aid kit in the cab. He left the back door unlocked for the repairmen. He mopped up the puddle from the leaky dishwasher, put down a flattened cardboard box on the still damp, ceramic tile floor, and set up an old box fan from the storage room on the cardboard to dry the wall, down which ran a metal conduit carrying electricity to the fire alarm box and the sprinkler system. He got out his step ladder and used a quick-dry spackle on the cracks in the kitchen walls. He was pretty much a one-man crew. Preferred fixing things himself—*old school*—whenever possible. The old box fan made too much noise to hear his radio, so he was stuck listening to the voice in his head calculating how long it had been since he'd last *gotten lucky*. He wasn't into this semi-celibate state to which Hannah—a truly good-looking woman, which made this all the more vexing—had moved them. But what options did he have? Divorce? He still loved the woman and certainly not while the kids were still in the house. Cheating? That would make him the bad guy. He didn't care for that role. Besides, it wasn't as if anyone else were interested in him these days. He figured his boyish good looks were a thing of the past. Or maybe he was just having some sort of mid-life crisis? Call Dr. Phil! Who the heck knew? When he got to the fire alarm wall, the old dishwasher had continued to leak under the cardboard. He got out the mop again, wiped up the water, and stood on the cardboard with the fan to keep from slipping on the damp, tile floor. But when he turned to spackle the corner of the wall, his elbow brushed the fire alarm box—*Bam!*—he heard himself yell—"Oh-h-h!"—as the electricity shot into his elbow, crossed through his chest, and continued down through his feet into the floor. As the power threw him suddenly backwards, his heart stopped—

and everything went black.

When he came to, he was on the floor, staring up at the ceiling—tingling head-to-toe—next to the leaky dishwasher. His heart beat again; he wasn't dead; his family would be all right. There was a ringing in his ears and the soles of his feet burned from the current that had escaped his body into the ceramic floor. But his ankle didn't hurt anymore. His elbow did though, as if someone had hit it with a hammer. He felt oddly at peace on the floor and so was in no hurry to get up. He heard voices, then two guys in green and gray work uniforms stood over him.

"Dude, are you all right?" the younger one with silver, stud earrings asked.

Mike sat up and calmly explained about the fan and the wet floor and the fire alarm box and his elbow, which was now circularly bruised where the electricity had entered his body.

The balding guy with the salt-and-pepper goatee checked the fan. "This old piece a' crap isn't even grounded. Cardboard's wet on the bottom. Looks like you became the ground, Buddy." He inspected the fire alarm box, too. "I wonder if this current is two-twenty?"

"If that was two-twenty," the younger guy surmised, "this son-of-a-bitch would be dead right now."

"No way," salt-and-pepper argued. "Two-twenty's a lot stronger, but the electrocution throws you. One-ten sticks you to the current. That's what kills you."

While the repairmen continued to argue voltage and whether or not Mike should be dead, he got up on his own.

They both looked at him. The ringing continued in his ears.

"Dude." The younger guy stared closely at him. "Your eyes are buggin' like light bulbs."

The goateed guy added: "And your hair's standing straight outta your head. Maybe we should take you to the hospital?"

Instead of going to the hospital, Mike took a walk. Down the street at the gas station mart, he purchased a can of Starbuck's Doubleshot—six-and-a-half ounces of espresso, cream, and sugar—from the refrigerated section. Shot it down. Went back to work and finished painting the kitchen in what seemed like no time. Got paid from Bill when he returned, who was more concerned about the accident. ("Really sorry you got electrocuted, Mike.") Drove to the bank, deposited the check in his business account, then home with cash in his wallet. Really didn't feel any worse for the wattage, which was what he told Hannah when he got there. She was making a salad in the kitchen. Both kids were eating dinner out with their friends.

"You got electrocuted?"

"Uh huh."

She stopped tearing the lettuce. "Are you all right? Did you go to the hospital?"

"Yes and no."

"What?"

"Yes, I'm all right. No, I didn't go to the hospital."

"My God." She came over and hugged him, then warned him like a mother: "Be careful, Babe."

He nodded.

She gave him a quick peck on the lips but stopped herself in mid-turn-away. "Oo. You're kind of... " She paused, trying to figure it out.

He offered: "Tingly?"

"Yeah. *Tingly.*"

"I've been this way ever since I was electrocuted."

"Huh?" She kissed him again, harder.

He took a quick shower (the beads of water crackled off his skin) and they rendezvoused in their bedroom just after dark. Talk about *getting lucky!* Sparks flew as they hadn't flown in years (if ever). They were great in bed that night. Hannah even said so: "Wow, that was great." She panted to get her breath back.

But he was invigorated—*electrified!* He felt as if he could make love all night. Or at least until ten o'clock when the kids were due home (school night). So they did.

The next morning, he was still tingly and his elbow was stiff. But his ankle didn't hurt at all. In fact, there was a spring in his step. And the ringing in his ears gradually morphed into an unceasing hum, with which he became quite comfortable.

Later that evening, his daughter complained from the den: "I hate this thing! It's too slow. We need a new computer!"

He was tired of hearing it. "Get out of the way." Alice got up and he sat down. The hourglass icon blinked intermittently next to the cursor arrow on the screen. "What are you trying to do?"

"Download some pictures for my term paper."

He stared at the blinking hour-glass, unsure of what to do. Hmm. He strummed his fingers along the keyboard frame, then suddenly, the hour-glass disappeared and the printer started printing.

Alice leaned over his shoulder. "What did you do?"

"Nothing. Just strummed the keyboard."

"Well, whatever you did, it's working." She moved him out of the chair, typed in some instructions, and the printer immediately churned out another picture. "Wow. This thing hasn't worked this fast in years. Thanks, Dad."

He nodded, unsure of what, if anything, he had done. But being the parent of teenagers, he was content to accept any credit one of them directed his way.

Hannah woke him that night to make love. It was great. The next night, too. They were suddenly like young lovers again who couldn't get enough of each other.

And because his ankle no longer hurt, he was able to get back to his every-other-day running regimen. He felt lighter and faster than he had in years, putting his mid-life crisis in the rear-view mirror. He even contemplated running in the L.A. Marathon again as he cruised painlessly along Colorado Boulevard early Sunday morning. The sun was already out but he had on a white cap and sleeveless tee, shades, and sunscreen, so the heat didn't bother him at all. In fact, the ultraviolet rays warming his body seemed to further invigorate him, like a solar panel absorbing energy, re-charging his already super-charged system. It was then that he saw her—

across the street, wearing the same cautionary-colored yellow singlet and red shorts—running about a half-block up ahead in the same direction as he. Hmm. He looked over his shoulder for traffic. When clear, he cut across the four opposing lanes, hopped the curb on the other side, and turned up the pace. He targeted the back of her yellow top as it bobbed up and down ahead of him. The target grew larger as he got nearer. He matched her step-for-step—but with more power per stride—so she didn't hear him gaining and didn't respond until he ran past her—without looking over—as they both leapt off the curb into the crosswalk at Lake Avenue. He was a step ahead when they hopped the curb on the other side and both continued to race east down Colorado Boulevard. He could feel her hanging closely. She had accepted the challenge and picked up her pace to match his. And why not? She had run away from him a few weeks ago like he was dead meat. Probably figured he couldn't keep up this pace for much longer. Could. Did. A mile later, she still hadn't caught him. And returning the favor, he didn't bother to look back, as he continued to pull away.

As usual, he stopped at the park for water. But as he bent-over the fountain and drank, from behind he heard footsteps approaching. It was her, breathing deeply, behind wrap-around shades. She, too, stopped for a drink, nodded hello. It was the first time they had seen each other face-to-face. Hers was likewise tanned from exercising in the sun, yet still smooth. Attractive. Late twenties, maybe early thirties. He nodded back and held on the water for her. She took a drink. "Mm. Thanks."

"Sure." He took another drink.

"You run well," she said.

"You, too."

It had been two weeks since he'd visited CD at Children's Hospital, where she had recently received her first chemo treatment. So he hopped the Gold Line to the Red Line and got off at Children's Hospital again. Took the stairs this time (good cardiovascular and endurance training) up to CD's floor. The pillows propped her up in the hospital bed. But she didn't look well—sort of pasty-pale— and didn't feel like talking. The captain's cap sat next to the paper mask on the nightstand. Her mother told him CD had vomited earlier after trying to eat. And that John had gone back to work but would be visiting later. One of them always stayed with her, so that she was never alone. He knew from visiting other people with chronic illnesses that sick people didn't always want visitors, and he felt as if he were intruding. He rambled on some more about the track team, then said his goodbyes, and promised to come back and see her again soon when she was feeling better. On the way out, he squeezed CD's big toe, which was under the covers, but held it this time for a little while longer. And this time, she smiled.

So he smiled, too. "Promise."

John called him that night from the hospital. "She's feeling much better since your visit. Perked right up. She was even able to keep a little food down at dinner. They're releasing her from the hospital tomorrow until her next chemo treatment. My wife wanted me to call and thank you. She said your visit was like a miracle."

And just like that, Mike the contractor, Mike the volunteer coach, Mike the computer repairman had suddenly graduated to become Mike the performer of minor miracles. He laughed to himself. *What next?* he thought. *What next?*

Sheree, the pony-tailed runner in yellow top and red shorts, ran with a local running club around the Rose Bowl every Thursday afternoon at five. At the water fountain, she had invited Mike to join her. Them. He told her he might. Thursday was his day to run and as it turned out, he finished his cabinet job early that afternoon. So he figured, *What the heck?* It wasn't as if he were going to join the club or anything. Just run with them. It had been a couple years since he'd run competitively with adults and he was anxious to see how well he matched-up now.

He drove his truck over to the Rose Bowl, parked on the street, and watched the unending stream of runners, walkers, dogs on leashes, bicyclists, parents pushing babies in streamlined strollers, and in-line skaters of all sizes, shapes, and colors, all ages, races, and levels, as they circled in both directions in opposing lanes at varying speeds. The fastest of all was the peloton—an elite group of fifty-or-so racing bicyclists, who sped past hunched-over their handlebars, creating with their mass the elongated shape of a pointed teardrop, ever-changing but continuously averaging 26-miles-per-hour. As the sounds of their sprockets and spokes whirred past, he spotted her pony tail in the midst of a group of runners in team red singlets, which she, too, wore with her red shorts. He locked his truck and with water bottle in hand, ran to catch up.

The road around the Rose Bowl and half of the golf course and the restaurant was 3.1 miles. The club runners, most of whom carried water bottles clipped to a belt or camel-backs with tubular drinking spouts, spread out according to their performance levels. He ran with Sheree, who was the fastest of the half-dozen women in the group. A few of the dozen or so men ran ahead of them. But Sheree seemed content to let them go.

"Don't let me hold you back," she said, without turning her head towards him.

"I'm fine." Admittedly, he was tempted to run down a couple of the young bucks ahead. He felt capable. His recent training was returning him to his pre-injury speed. He was able to stay out for miles longer on his runs. And he had his kick back, too. Next time, maybe he would challenge the younger leaders?

But Coach Mike's Ferris wheel ride had crested. Because halfway through their second lap—as the peloton whirred past once again—he felt an ever-so-slight twinge in his ankle. It wasn't much. He half-convinced himself it was just his imagination, as they continued south past the restaurant parking lot. But by the time they approached his parked truck a quarter-mile south, the damn ache in his damn ankle was back again.

"That's it for me." He didn't want to do any more damage.

"Oh." Sheree seemed surprised as she looked over. "Okay. See you next week?"

"Maybe." He slowed and stopped across from his truck,

watched her ponytail bob side-to-side as she ran away, without looking back.

By the time he got home it was dusk and he was limping. Hannah opened the door.

"Not your ankle again?"

He nodded.

She kissed him hello. "Huh?"

"What?"

She kissed him again, harder, stopped. "It's gone."

"What?"

"You know. The *tingle*."

It was then that he noticed the hum in his ears—to which he'd become so comfortably accustomed—had also ceased.

She lamented: "I guess we both knew it couldn't last forever."

He nodded, "Yeah," and hobbled to the kitchen for a bag of ice.

Later that night, Hannah turned him down. And pretty much put him on notice for any future advances: "Look, Mister. You've gotten lucky enough in the last three weeks to last the next three months. Personally, I'm satiated. So stay on your own side of the bed." She pushed him away.

He rolled over in the dark and lay on his back. Reminiscing the recent good times, he tried to ignore the pain in his ankle. Eventually, he fell off to sleep.

Admittedly, he was depressed for the next week or so.

His ankle ached. Couldn't run. Not even on the track at practice with his team. ("Come on, Coach Mike. Hurry up!") To stay in shape, he lifted weights and rode the stationary bike in their garage. But spinning endlessly in the same stupid place just wasn't his thing. He remembered reading a long time ago how Bruce Lee—the '70s martial artist and action movie hero—used to electrocute himself with doses of low voltage before his work-outs to super-charge his system into an elevated state, where reflexes became instantaneous and side-kicks a blur. Of course, Mr. Lee died of a heart attack at the age of 33. Remembering how his own heart had seized in his chest when the electricity passed through it, he figured the two facts might be related. But who knew? Maybe Bruce Lee liked red meat and his heart condition was congenital? Either way, Mike figured it was his own good fortune that he'd popped those two aspirins for his ankle before his accidental electrocution. Might've saved his life. Just dumb luck.

He was having a heck of a time figuring out what to buy Hannah for their anniversary. Because it was their twentieth, he wanted to get her something special, but she didn't like him to spend a lot of money on her. (She was great that way.) But still, he had to come up with something good and soon. So one night after work, he went to Old Town to window-shop (for what he didn't know) outside the boutiques. He tried not to limp like an old man even though his ankle complained about every step on the unforgiving sidewalk, when the cellphone rang in his pocket. He stopped and answered:

"Hello?"

"Mike? This is Bill at Marten's. That stupid dishwasher leaked again and flooded that last wall you painted. I have the repairman here right now. So I need you to paint it again. Health inspector's coming next week."

"We have to dry it out first. I'm just down the street from you right now. I'll stop by on my way home."

When he got to the restaurant, it was already closed for the night. He went through the back door. The kitchen help were already gone. The water was already mopped up and the same old box fan was set-up on another flattened cardboard box—just like before—blowing on the lower portion of the wall, where the drywall was swollen and the paint bubbled with moisture. *De ja voux*. Step on the wet cardboard. Touch the fire alarm box. Wham! Bam! *Electrified* again! He laughed to himself. Heck of an anniversary present for Hannah. (Him, too!) But of course, he wasn't going to electrocute himself for sex. Not even great sex. Lots of really great sex. And a pain-free ankle, so he could run again. But that was too damn crazy even for him—mid-life crisis or not. He didn't need Dr. Phil to figure that out. A different repairman—middle-aged and mustachioed, in the same company uniform—closed his toolbox next to the culprit dishwasher.

"You the contractor?"

Mike nodded.

"You the guy who got electrocuted?"

He laughed and nodded again. "One and the same."

"Must've been a hell of a trip."

"Yeah. You have no idea."

"That two-oh-eight really packs a wallop."

"'Two-oh-eight?'"

The repairman nodded knowingly. "It's a special current, special circuit. So if all the other circuits burn-out in a fire," he pointed to the metal conduit protecting the wires leading to the fire alarm box on the wall, "the sprinkler system still activates. That's its sole purpose."

Sole purpose? Mike glanced to the heavens, but mostly remembered how the bottoms of his feet had burned as the *two-oh-eight* passed through his *soles* into the tile floor. The cellphone rang in his pocket again. "Excuse me." He stepped into the empty hallway. "Hello?"

It was John, CD's dad. They were down at the hospital. CD had just gone through another session of chemo. She was sick. And to complicate matters, in all their moving from the hospital to home and back again, they had somehow lost the captain's cap the team had given her. "I hate to ask, Coach. But could you get her another cap? She feels really bad from the chemo. We thought it might cheer her up. Like the last time you visited."

Mike said sure. They talked a little more. He hung up, slipped the phone back into the pocket of his Levi's.

Bill came in the back door. "Stupid dishwasher. How soon can you re-paint?"

"Soon as it dries out. Leave the fan on overnight. I'll stop by tomorrow."

The repairman walked out of the kitchen, handed Bill another bill.

"It better be fixed this time," Bill said. "We don't want Mike here electrocuting himself again."

Repairman number three explained: "It's an old machine. You fix one thing, something else breaks."

Number three exited out the back door; Bill went up front; and Mike went back in the kitchen to make sure the fan was pointed where it was most needed. He'd call and order another cap for CD. But it wasn't the cap that had made her feel better—*Like the last time you visited*—when he'd promised her he'd come back. He adjusted the fan. But when he turned around, from under the old dishwasher, a tiny trickle of water started to inch its way down the mortared joint of the ceramic tile towards the flattened cardboard under the fan. In the doorway, Bill asked on his way out: "Got it under control?"

But instead of reporting the new leak, in front of which he stood, blocking Bill's view, Mike turned around and asked: "You have any aspirin?"

"Sure. Medicine cabinet in the ladies' bathroom. Ankle again?" He tossed the extra set of keys to Mike again.

"What else?"

"Don't forget to set the alarm. Thanks for fixing things. See you tomorrow." On his way out the back door, Bill added: "Hope it feels better."

"Yeah. Me, too." But Bill was already gone and didn't hear him. Didn't matter. He put the keys in his pocket, got two aspirins from the ladies' bathroom, and washed them down with a water bottle from the big refrigerator in the kitchen, then stood staring down at his feet, where the trickle of water once again ran under the flattened cardboard under the ungrounded fan under the fire alarm box on the wall. Hmm. *Like the last time you visited*. He'd promised her.

He took a deep breath. What the heck? It would be over before he knew it.

MARK BARKAWITZ

ROMENICO'S PIZZA

I'd just finished my first cycle of chemo. I'd been misdi-
agnosed for the past nine months, so I was already stage-
three. And with multiple myeloma, there is no stage-four.
As my recently-referred oncologist Dr. Hu had explained:
"You're already dead." So my survival was definitely *iffy*.
And with a broken back from the cancer in my blood and
bones—every bone in my body—I was extremely uncom-
fortable and weak. In fact, I needed a wheeled-walker just to
get around the house and back yard. But mostly, I gobbled
Vicodin and squirmed in the recliner in my bedroom, trying
to find a comfortable position for my unstable spine, passing
the time in a haze in front of the TV or trying to read. Com-
prehension? Forget about it. My cellphone rang.

"Hello?"

"Mark? Thank God. It's Frank."

"Hey, Frankie." Frank and I had been good friends since
grade school at St. Philip the Apostle School in Pasadena.
He'd been the drummer in one of our teenage, garage bands,

The Bitter Ends. He still played on Sundays in a Christian rock band at his church. I kidded him that the drummer gig was the reason he'd been *born-again*. He lived out of town now but already knew I was sick from our last phone conversation a month ago. "What's up, Bro?"

"Uh, well, I-I don't want to upset you. But..."

I half-laughed. "But what?" My diagnosis had caused me a lot of grief and anger. I was trying to get past that now to a more positive state of mind, which I knew would aid in my recovery—*if* recovery were even possible. Admittedly, it had been an up-and-down struggle so far.

"Well, I was just up at Romenico's on my way through town." It was a long-time, family-owned, Italian restaurant. "And Ronnie's been telling people you're already dead." Ronnie Romenico was one of the owners, who still worked in the kitchen he and his brothers had inherited from their father.

"What?" I sat up in the recliner, which felt like a knife in my back. Ronnie had also been a childhood friend—of sorts. My little brother had been the starting second baseman on a Little League all-star team, until Ronnie's father showed up with pizzas for the whole team and its coaches. Next practice, Ronnie—who was shaped more like one of his father's meatballs back then—was the starting second baseman and my little brother was on the bench. "That son-of-a—!"

"Yeah. That's why I was relieved when you answered the phone. He said both you and Mike Alessi had died a couple weeks ago." Mike was another mutual, childhood friend, who *had* actually died recently from throat cancer—damn cigarettes—and whose funeral was two weeks past. I hadn't gone because of my appearance and the walker. I didn't want everyone thinking—*He'll be next*—about me. And I sure as heck didn't want someone starting a rumor that I was already dead! I had a lot of friends in this town and Romenico's had a lot of customers. That darn Ronnie already had me in my grave and was kicking in the dirt!

"I swear to God if I had the energy, I'd go up there right now and give him hell!" But I didn't have the energy. And I looked like hell.

A year later, I was recovering from spine-fusion surgery. Piece 'a cake compared to my cancer treatments—six months of chemotherapy and a stem cell transplant at City of Hope—which had successfully obliterated all the cancer from my system. (Thank God for medical insurance!) My back was still a bit sensitive and I moved cautiously but otherwise felt great! I'd dumped the wheeled-walker and prescription pain pills. A couple ibuprofens were all I needed for my occasional pain. It was like a miracle—an extremely slowly developing miracle. It was Friday night and my wife didn't cook on Friday nights after working all week. So she asked me:

"Want to order a pizza for dinner?"

"Sure, sounds good."

She took out her cellphone. "Pietro's?"

It was just a few blocks from our house. And they made good pies. But not tonight. "No. Romenico's. Call it in. I'll pick it up."

"Is your back okay to drive?"

"Yep."

Another mutual, high school friend of ours had once said of Ronnie: "He makes good pizzas, but he doesn't think his shit stinks." I had to laugh. I knew what he meant. I parked at the curb just up the street from Romenico's and climbed carefully out of my truck cab. As I walked towards the restaurant, I wasn't sure what I was going to say to Ronnie, but figured I had to say something. I'd been quite confrontational as a young man, but had mellowed considerably over the years, especially after my bout with The Grim Reaper. Live and let live. So who knew? I went into the take-out side of the restaurant. There were only two other customers ahead of me. I gave my phone order and paid the teenage girl working the cash register behind the take-out counter. When she gave me my change and the medium, vegetarian pizza in its large, flat box, I asked:

"Is Ronnie working tonight?"

"Big Ronnie or Little Ronnie?"

"*Old* Ronnie."

"Oh, uh, yeah." She looked at me uncertainly. "He's in the kitchen."

I smiled, "Could you tell him Mark Barkawitz is here?" and dropped a couple bucks in the tip jar on the counter.

"Sure." She walked to the end of the short hall, turned to the kitchen, and I could see her lips moving as she spoke to someone off-stage, so to speak, then pointed towards me. A few seconds later, Ronnie's head leaned out from the kitchen into the hallway, staring uncertainly in my direction. He continued to stare, frowning, then stepped out into the hallway and walked slowly towards me, wiping his hands on his apron, his mouth gaped open, as if he were seeing a ghost. It was all I could do to keep from cracking-up. But I didn't laugh.

"Hey, Ronnie. Been a while." I smiled and reached my hand over the counter.

He shook it uncertainly. "Yeah. How you doing, Mark?"

"Just had a little back surgery. But other than that," I was still smiling, "I feel like a million bucks." My cancer treatments, surgeries, and stem cell transplant had cost nearly that much.

"Yeah. Yeah. You look good."

For a dead guy, I figured he figured.

"You, too, Ronnie." And he did: just a little older, grayer, and trimmed-down to his proper size. "Well, I better get rolling before your pizza gets cold. Say hi to your brothers for me. Good seeing you again." Sometimes saying less was more.

"Yeah. Yeah. You, too, Mark." He headed back towards the kitchen, looking back at me once, then again, just to reassure himself, I suppose. I could only imagine what he told the kitchen help.

"Damn, this is good pizza," I told my wife, before taking another slice.

"Um hm," she agreed, swallowed. "Did you see your friend Ronnie up there?"

"Yep." I couldn't help smiling, remembering his bewildered expression when he saw me at the counter, as if risen from my grave and born again. I took another bite of his pizza and gobbled it down. Who knew recovery was going to be this much fun?

A HAPPY GUY

I'm usually a pretty happy guy. I was even happy the day my spine was sliced open and hardware installed. Of course, I woke-up with a morphine-strength drip and the ability to self-administer every ten minutes. (The nurses took away that toy the next day.) Still, I was happy.

But admittedly, the cancer that had spawned in my marrow—weakening my vertebrae, threatening my life—really ticked me off. I wanted to kick cancer's butt—break its back, just as it had mine! But anger and machismo aren't enough against such a ruthless killer.

It's been said it takes a village to raise a child. I know it took my HMO, primary-care physician, two great oncologists, talented and caring nurses, office staff, and the City of Hope to raze the cancer from my blood and bones, then their top-notch neurosurgeon to screw my back together again— one incredibly lucky, grateful, and happy guy!

MARK BARKAWITZ

AMPHIBIOUS AGAIN

Doheny Beach, July 9, 2012—Just got out of the ocean. One year ago last summer, I was in an isolation unit at City of Hope getting a stem cell transplant to wipe-out the cancer that had broken my L-5 vertebra and threatened my life. Five-months-and-one-week after spine-fusion surgery— three titanium rods installed with a half-dozen screws by world-class neurosurgeon Dr. Rahul Jandial—I strapped my surfboard to the roof racks on my truck and drove down anxiously. (I was supposed to wait six months but I'd been working-out vigorously, swimming laps so I wouldn't drown, and it was over 100 degrees in Pasadena!)

I was able to paddle-out. But I never *really* knew for sure if I'd actually be able to surf again, a sport which I'd taken up as a teenager and had continued all of my adult life until my back broke from the cancer 2½ years ago. There was a small, south swell running—perfect, little waves for my liquid re-hab. I caught three, small waves—muscle-memory took over as soon as I rode each—and then paddled-in. Didn't want to overdo it on my first day back out. Rock-danced the shallows to the sandy shore. Tomorrow, I'd return and ride six, small waves.

Sitting on the warm sand under a clear, baby-blue sky, staring out at kindred surfers bobbing like multi-colored corks on the blue-green ocean, I pounded my chest, thanking all—All—who had helped return me to this pantheistic altar, at peace with the majestic world around me, a small part of something much bigger. *Cowabunga, Brah!* There was life after cancer; and it was good!

DESTINY'S STEPCHILD

"Have you started working again?" my oncologist Dr. Hu asked, as he stared at the monitor, studying my blood work-up from my most recent donation at LabCorp.

"I have," I proudly replied, sitting on the examination table, my feet dangling above the floor. I'd been down almost 2½ years with a broken back and the incurable bone and blood cancer that had caused it. I'd survived financially off Disability payments (Thank God for Social Security!) and my dwindling savings accounts. And luckily, my wife worked, too.

"Just got a job with the Sierra Madre Grocery Company. I'm their new Quality Control man." It was mostly driving the freeways from store-to-store—negotiating L.A.'s worst-in-the-nation traffic jams—doing inventory, re-stocking the items on their personal shelves. One week—I was still in my trial period with the company—and I already hated it. Specifically, the traffic jams and threat of road rage (mine), but I was glad to be physically-able to work again.

Staring behind his metal-framed glasses at the monitor, Dr. Hu asked: "I thought you were a contractor?" We'd come to know each other somewhat personally through the course of my treatments.

"I am. But I can't go back to that again."

"Why not?"

"You know—all the chemicals and pollutants in the paints and solvents and concrete dust and everything else. I almost killed myself once with that crud." On 10/8/'10, I was diagnosed with stage-three, multiple myeloma. My kidneys had shut down, and without treatment, I was told I would die in two days on 10/10/'10. The date still had an ominous ring to it. "Can't take a chance on doing that again."

"This all looks good," he said, still gazing at my computer-generated results. "Cell count's normal and not a trace of cancer in your system. M-spike's still there on your kidneys, but that's normal. It doesn't usually go away." Then he looked away from the monitor and at me. "Your cancer wasn't environmentally-caused."

"What? What do you mean?"

"There was a mark on your DNA, like a time-bomb, set to go off when it finally did."

"You mean I was destined to die at a specific time in my life from multiple myeloma since the day I was born?"

He was tall and stood over me on the examination table. "Since the day you were *conceived*."

"Whoa." I'd never really believed in *Destiny*—that our lives were fated—preordained by the gods, as the Vikings had believed, in the great mead hall of Valhalla that was their heaven. I was more a proponent of self-determination—that we made our own destinies by our actions. But only to a degree, of course. Sometimes, man couldn't overcome his physical surroundings.

"You're a lucky man," Dr. Hu said, a sly smile on his face. "See you again in three months."

A lucky man? I couldn't help smiling, as I drove my truck home from my check-up. I'd been told that before by others. And it was true. My life hadn't been charmed—I'd worked hard for what I had—but even the bad stuff had a way of righting itself eventually—and usually—for the better. Of course, I sure as heck hadn't *felt lucky* while going through six months of chemo, a stem cell transplant, and spine-fusion surgery. But if I had to get an incurable cancer—and apparently I did—it was lucky indeed I got one that was *treatable*. As a self-determinist, I'd previously-defined *luck* as *preparation meets opportunity*. But as a former third-baseman, I knew a hard-hit ground ball could take a bad hop and eat me up no matter how much I'd prepared.

I was truly glad to learn that I hadn't nearly-caused my own demise. So I never went back to work again for the Sierra Madre Grocery Company. Instead, I put the magnetic signs back on my truck that advertised my contracting business. The phone started ringing again. But I only worked locally now, staying off the freeways as much as possible. Cancer had a way of making you look at things differently. I didn't know how much time I had left, but I sure wasn't going to waste it immobilized in traffic jams, *raging* at my fellow drivers. Dr. Hu had originally gauged my survival in the two-to-five-years range. But as I'd recovered more fully, he opined at one of my check-ups:

"If we get you to five, we'll get you to ten. Then we'll cure you."

I was betting on it—*Luck* to trump *Destiny*. My ante was already sitting on the table. But I was in no hurry to play-out my hand. Life was good again. Valhalla could wait.

29 AGAIN

"Darn it." I'd just turned onto a side street and into a construction zone. Traffic was backed up with a flagman letting cars one-at-a-time past the open hole in the street, around which a half-dozen county workers stood watching one of their own in the hole with a shovel. As I waited in line in my car, I happened to gaze down a driveway at the end of which sat another old house partially-hidden in back by trees and bushes—a single-story stucco badly in need of a paint job—that looked somehow familiar. But I was waved through by the flagman before I could recognize the old place.

A few days later, I was in the same general vicinity. (I'd recently sold my business—a profitable travel and adventure agency—and was a semi-retired consultant now with no immediate need to be anywhere.) So just for the heck of it, I turned again onto Poppy Way, the same side street. The repair work had been completed—a freshly asphalted patch filled-in the hole in the street—with only parked cars at the curb. I stopped in the street where I had days earlier and again stared down the driveway at the old, stucco house in back. It had a distinctive, if somewhat confusing architectural design, with the steep roof of an English Tudor, the wood-framed windows and front porch of a California bungalow, and the knock-down stucco of a Spanish *casa*. Then it struck me:

"No, it can't be!"

In the waning years of my bachelorhood thirty-some years ago, I'd rented one side of an old duplex near the university. I'd heard it was going to be razed after I moved out—replaced by a condominium complex—but I'll be darned if that wasn't the same, old house! A car honked behind me in the street, so I drove away.

When my wife got home from work, I told her about seeing my former rental.

"Really? I thought they'd demolished that old place long ago." Anna was five years younger than I and still quite attractive: big brown eyes with a long and lean body firmed from rigorous, morning work-outs before work. I'd first spotted her on a campus tennis court thirty-some years ago—*Now there's a young lady with whom I could spend the rest of my life!*—and happily put my bachelor ways to rest. Hadn't been with another woman since.

"Apparently not. Guess they moved it instead."

"That old dump? Why on earth would anyone go to all that trouble?"

Funny, I didn't remember it as a *dump*. Just an old house that had been separated down the middle by a plaster wall to form two, rental units. Of course, my memories of the old place were quite different than hers. For me, it had been my *bachelor pad* from a time when my life was very different. I'd lived there the years that I attended the university. I was bartending back then at a local nightclub (Talk about *adventure!*) and worked-out regularly—lifting weights and hitting the heavy-bag—in the gym next door. So between college and work, I met a lot of young co-eds and bar foxes. Admittedly, I took advantage of my trappings: study, work-out, work, party; study, work-out, work, party. (Not always in that order.) It was the kind of grind that only a young man could survive for any length of time. Right up to the time I married my wife (one of the co-eds) and we bought a house just a few miles away, where we raised two kids, who were both away at college themselves now.

I couldn't get the old place out of my head. So the next day—I didn't have much to do—I parked at the curb on Poppy Way and got out. But as I walked down the driveway, a middle-aged woman in a baggy T-shirt and sweat pants stood on the front porch, sweeping. And that woman looked exactly like Rose, the old lady—heck, I was her age now—who'd lived next door to me in the other half of the duplex!

"Rose?"

She looked up from her sweeping, smiled as she recognized me. "Hi, Honey." She'd always called me *Honey*. I'm not sure it wasn't because she couldn't remember my name was Marty, even though we were such close neighbors. She'd had a few brain surgeries, which had left her *a little ditsy*, as her husband Al had put it.

"Rose. My God, it is you! You haven't changed a bit." And she hadn't, from the crow's feet at the outsides of her full face right down to her old house slippers. She had to be nearly ninety now but didn't look a day over sixty! How?

"Thanks, Honey." She leaned on her broom handle and stared down at me from the porch. "Can't say the same for you though. Heh-heh," she cackled. She'd always been brutally honest. Al had said she couldn't lie *'cause a' the brain thing*. "But ya' never know," she added.

Never know what? "Did you find the Fountain of Youth or something? You look great!"

"Or somethin'," she agreed, cackled again, went back to her sweeping. Someone coughed inside her side of the old duplex—a hacking from the past.

"My God, that can't be Al in there?"

"Can. Is. Still smokin' those damn cigarettes." It was the only time she ever swore. "Still keepin' me up at night with his coughin'." She stopped sweeping, leaned on the broom handle again, and looked at me for sympathy. "You know how long I been out on that couch in the livin' room, tryin' ta get some sleep?"

Yes, I did know how long—47 years! The walls of the duplex were thin plaster, so Al's nightly coughing attacks had also awakened me long ago. Al had been 71 or 84 or 67, depending on how he felt when I asked him. He'd had lung cancer for seventeen years back then! Had been given a year to live. Had instead buried three doctors. (Or so he'd claimed.) Smoked two-packs-a-day—Camels, no filters. So how? How?

"Rose, are you telling me Al's still alive, too?"

But the coughing from inside the duplex answered for her. "That's why we bought the place, Honey. Good seein' ya' again. Next time, don't take so long ta come back." She opened the aluminum screen door that I'd long-ago helped Al in his undershirt install; all the while a burning Camel had drooped loosely from the corner of his lips. She closed the door.

"What the—?" I wasn't sure what to do. I wanted some answers. I walked up on the porch, was going to knock, but even with the door closed, could hear Al's hacking inside. This was crazy. How? Instead, I rang the doorbell on my side of the duplex. Nothing. I opened the old, aluminum screen door and knocked on the familiar, Hulk-green-painted front door. Nothing. I checked; it was locked. I tried looking in through the windows but the curtains were pulled closed. Hey, weren't those my old curtains? One of my old (young then) girlfriends before Anna had sewn them for me. So I couldn't see inside. And I couldn't help looking back—I don't know how many times—as I walked away.

When Anna got home from work, I told her about my day.

"Rose and Al are still alive? That's remarkable." She put down her school stuff on the dining room table, sat, sighed, worn from a long day of teaching and parent conferences.

"*Remarkable?* It's downright eerie. Rose hasn't aged a day. Not another wrinkle on her face. And I swear to God, she was wearing the same old pair of house slippers!"

"What are you getting so worked up about? So they're

alive. Wonders of modern medicine. People are living longer these days." She sighed again. "Listen, Hon. I have to make up a lesson plan for tomorrow." She didn't need to say more.

The next day, I went down to City Hall—I didn't have diddly to do anyway—and had a clerk look up the address of my old house in the city records.

"Hm." She didn't look over at me from behind her eyeglasses as she squinted at the monitor on her desk for more information. "There's a condominium complex there now. Wait a minute. You're right. There was a small house there years ago. Built in nineteen-oh-three. It was scheduled to be razed thirty years ago, but the city declared it a historical monument and ordered it moved to another lot. Maybe I can find out where?"

I already knew *where*.

"You did what?" Anna was late getting home from work. She put down the bag of groceries in the kitchen. "Don't you have anything better to do with your time?"

I didn't.

"*Historical monument*," she scoffed. "You need a hobby."

That night as I slept restlessly—adventuring back in my dreamscape to another time, another place—it suddenly occurred to me and I woke with a start: "The key!"

"What?" I'd woken Anna. "Are you all right?"

"The key. Remember?" I sat up in the dark. "I used to stash one outside in the fuse box. It might still be there."

"Honey, you're driving me crazy with this stupid, old house stuff. What does it matter? Go to sleep. I have to work in the morning, you know." But she didn't pose it like a question, instead yanking the covers and rolling away from me.

I knew. And I knew what I had to do.

The next day, I was up early—Anna had been gone for an hour already—grabbed a cup of coffee, drove down, parked on Poppy Way, and walked down the long drive-way, sipping my coffee. In back, the whirly-sprinkler from thirty years ago attached to the hose watered the small patch of grass out front but Rose wasn't outside. I didn't hear Al either. I went around to the back of the house to the fuse box and pulled open its metal door. Inside were the anti-quated, glass fuses of a knob-and-tube electrical system guarded by a spider's web, and in a dusty box of spare fuses, the key to my former front door!

I slipped the key into the lock. At first it didn't want to move—atrophied from years of non-use—then it turned to the right and the lock clicked open. I pushed open the door and stepped inside.

"Whoa."

The darkened room looked just as it had thirty years ago when I moved out. Because it was slated to be razed, I'd abandoned most of my old furnishings—Anna and I had gotten new furniture from our families as wedding gifts—figuring it'd all go to the dump with the rest of the house af-ter Rose had let in the Goodwill people to take what they wanted. (Anna and I had been on our honeymoon, snorkeling in Tahiti.) I sipped my still warm coffee, traveling back in time. The flowered curtains that my girlfriend Cassidy had sewn for me, the wall-to-wall royal blue carpeting, the 19-inch black & white TV with broken rabbit ears and questionable horizontal hold, and the Mediterranean corner sofa I'd gotten at a yard sale, on which I'd wooed co-eds and bar foxes alike, hoping to persuade them farther into my bachelor lair. Even the old stereo with the turntable was still in the corner. I pressed the power button; it lit on. The turntable started revolving, the needle arm lifted automatically, swung slowly over the album that I'd apparently forgotten on it thirty years ago and lowered the needle somewhere (it hadn't been very accurate; one of the many reasons I'd left it behind) onto the black vinyl, which scratched loudly over the two, plywood speakers (also yard sale acquisitions) at opposite ends of the room. It began in the middle: "*Welcome to the Hotel California,*" the Eagles invited. I turned down the volume, blew a dust cloud off the LP, coughed, and stepped away. The scratchy soundtrack of my past and Cassidy's flowered curtains covering the windows cornered me on two sides. She was the most-alluring of the female clientele who'd frequented my shifts at the club: a dark-haired beauty with alabaster skin, baby-blue eyes, and full breasts, which she accentuated with cleavage-baring tops. I'd met her on a full-moon-Saturday-night (always trouble in an alcohol-enhanced environment), when a drunken ex-boyfriend grabbed her ass. I went over the bar like a pommel horse—I was young then, strong and cock-sure of myself—and directed him physically out the door. From that night on, she was my *main squeeze*—a term from the past that suddenly popped into my head—for the next year-and-a-half.

I started down the long, narrow hallway, looked in at the kitchen—its bare walls and old, linoleum floor a yellowing time-capsule. But it was the bedroom at the end of the hall that I entered.

"Whoa," I repeated.

My old waterbed sat where I'd left it. The bluish vinyl was collapsed flatly—I'd emptied the water with a hose out the window—with thirty years of dust blanketing it now. I couldn't help laughing. Wow, did I put that thing to use! But not all the memories were good. The so-called *carefree* bachelor life was actually strife with emotional entanglements. That was where Cassie and I had parted ways. The old plaster walls were scarred with nails that had hung pictures and cracks from the shifting foundation. I pushed open the bathroom door. The morning sunlight leaned in through the cloudy glass at the window over the claw-footed tub which took most of the tiled floor space in the small room. I'd spent hours soaking, reading texts, relaxing in that white porcelain tub. But when I turned to the medicine cabinet over the sink, the face in the cloudy mirror that stared back at me was me—thirty years ago! No lines, no wrinkles, and a full head of beach-boy-blond hair! I dropped my coffee cup, which spilled and broke on the tile floor around my sneakered feet, and watched my smooth mouth gape open in the dusty, veined mirror. How? How?

"What are you saying?" Anna asked, eyeing me like one of her young pupils who had concocted a whopper. "That you somehow magically turned twenty-nine again when you stepped inside your old house?"

"That's what I'm saying. I know, I know it sounds crazy. But I swear to God I'm not making it up!"

"Oh, Honey." She sat at the dining room table with her purse and school work. I'd barely let her in the front door before accosting her with my news. "What do you want me to say? That can't have happened. You know that. Don't you?"

"In my head yes. But if you'd seen me in that mirror…"

"And then you changed back?"

"As soon as I stepped off the porch. I watched my hands age. My face, too, when I checked the rear view mirror back at the car."

She nodded, pursed her lips. I wasn't sure what she was going to say next. I don't think she knew either. So I offered:

"Come down there with me."

She sighed. "I have a job. I have mid-term grades to get out. I don't have time for this nonsense. Don't you have any work to do?"

"Nothing pressing." I really didn't. I was a travel and adventure consultant with no one to consult, nowhere to go, and nothing to do. "And you're the one who told me to get a hobby. Remember?"

"Honey, this is not a *hobby*. It's becoming an obsession. Do you understand the difference?"

After dinner, I drove down and parked on Poppy Way with Anna. It was evening. We walked down the driveway together. When she got a good look at the old place—Rose wasn't out front and their door was closed—she stopped.

"Oh, my goodness. It is your old house."

"See, I told you. Come on, the key's around back."

I took her by the hand and led her around to the back of the house, where we retrieved the key from the old box of fuses in the fuse box where I'd replaced it after my first visit. On the front porch, I slipped it into the lock, when from behind, a man's voice ordered:

"Hold it a minute."

When we looked around, a buff, young policeman in short sleeves stood behind us in the driveway. His right hand rested on his holstered weapon. His other held a flashlight that wasn't yet on.

"Do you live here?"

"I used to." I didn't mention when.

"But not now?"

"No, not now. This side is empty. Except for some of my old stuff."

"Step off the porch, please."

We did. Showed him our I.D.s and I made up an excuse about what we were doing there without the *magical* part so I didn't sound crazy. He explained that the neighbor in the front house had called-in a complaint about a stranger—me?—snooping around the back house recently. So the police had been on the lookout.

"So you have a key?" he asked.

"I do." I didn't tell him from where I'd gotten it for fear he'd take it from me.

"Open the door," he ordered and followed us in. I turned on the light switch.

"Oh my goodness," Anna remarked. "It's just like it was thirty years ago!" She looked from one corner of the room to another.

"See, I told you."

Then she remembered: "But you look the same, Hon."

"What? Oh." I looked at the backs of my knuckled hands at the loose skin of a middle-aged man approaching the end of middle-age. "Huh?"

We followed the policeman who flipped on the flashlight and walked down the dark hallway, checking the nearly dark kitchen, and then into the bedroom. Again, I flipped on the light switch.

"Oh my goodness," Anna repeated, hiding her smile. "Your old waterbed."

"Yeah. Crazy, huh?" I had nothing but good memories with Anna in there.

The young, muscular policeman stuck his head in the bathroom, using the flashlight. "Okay. I think we're done in here." Apparently, he hadn't found any corpses, so we were exonerated.

"Wait a minute." I walked past him into the bathroom. But when I looked in the mirror in the gray light, I looked back at me. Anna's face entered the framed reflection behind me. I didn't need to turn on the light. She hadn't changed either.

I was losing it. That was the best way to explain it. There was really no other plausible explanation—I was losing it. Too much time on my hands. I needed to go back to work again or something. Advertise my availability. I didn't sleep well that night. Anna leaned over the bed and kissed me goodbye the next morning. But I just lay there for a while. There was no explaining what had happened. I made breakfast, then put on my shorts and sneaks and sunglasses and went for a walk. A long walk. As we'd left the old duplex last night, the cop knocked on Rose and Al's door, but they hadn't answered. I'd looked back as we walked up the driveway in the early darkness and thought I saw someone peeking between the curtains of their front window. Eventually on my walk that morning, I found myself drawn to Poppy Way again, staring down the driveway at my old house in back. I had to know.

I still had the key with me from last night. But as I slipped it into the lock, the other front door on the porch opened. Rose stood behind the screen door.

"We knew you'd be back again, Honey."

"Yeah. I mean. What's going on, Rose?"

"It don't work with new folk." Somewhere behind her, Al coughed and hacked. "Will ya' knock it off?" she yelled back into the apartment.

"What do you mean?"

"Heh, heh," she cackled. "That's why we kept it vacant for ya' all these years, Honey. Y'er furniture, too." She cackled again and closed the door.

"Wait a minute." But she didn't. Huh? I looked at the backs of my hands. The skin was tight. I went inside my old apartment, hurried down the hallway, through my bedroom, and into the bathroom. There in the dusty mirror, I stared back at me—29 again! Oh. My. God!

So the old house became my *obsession*, all right. I tried to get Anna to come back, explaining how the young cop's presence had broken *the spell* or whatever it was that enabled me—us?—to travel back in time, un-aging thirty years. But she refused. Threatened to have me *institutionalized if I didn't stop it!* So I had to lie to her about going back there. I bought a set of used clubs off Craigslist and told her I'd taken up golf as my new *hobby*.

But really, I spent most of my days in my old apartment. Rose and I became close neighbors like before. I started paying rent (same $165 a month as thirty years ago). She didn't have a spare key, so there was only the one in the fuse box for me, which she warned me not to duplicate. I asked questions; she replied cryptically. I'd always figured her word games were a result of *the brain thing*. She implied it best not to bring new stuff into the old environment. So I dug up a stack of old, scratched albums—soundtracks from my past in the duplex—from down in our basement at home and brought them back inside the apartment. Cleaned up the place with my old canister vacuum (another student era, yard sale deal) and worn broom still in the hall closet. Boiled water in the old, tea pot and made instant coffee from a half-filled jar of freeze-dried Folgers Crystals still in the cabinet that never went lower than half-empty. Filled and made-up the waterbed, just in case I slept over. Or *got lucky* again! I laughed to myself. I liked being 29 again. Did push-ups and crunches on the royal blue carpeting, flexing my newly-found, young-man muscles. Stared at myself in the bathroom mirror—*Damn, you're looking good!*—which I cleaned with an old bottle of Windex from under the sink. I took long, hot, soaking baths in the tub—admiring my sculptured abs—while Bruce Springsteen rasped loudly from the old speakers about his roving heart and Al hacked on the other side of the plaster wall, spitting in the face of cancer, flushing it down the toilet. But I soon grew bored with my new/old domain. I was the successor to Ponce de Leon and needed to share my Fountain-of-Youth adventure with someone. Someone from my past. Or it wouldn't work.

"How's your game coming?" Anna asked when I got home.

I'd stayed longer than I'd meant to. I wasn't sure what she meant. *"Game?"*

"Your golf game. You've been playing a lot lately. Haven't you?"

"Oh. Yeah. Uh, it's okay. I've been thinking about taking a lesson," I lied.

"Lessons are good," she agreed. But of course, she was a teacher.

The next day, I was back at my old place again. Blew the dust off a Boston album and put it on the turntable. They advised me: *"Don't look back."* But how could I not in my present surroundings? I got out the canister vacuum to clean up a little—I was just killing time really—put on the nozzle attachment for hand-held use, removed the couch cushions, and started sucking dirt and crumbs from thirty years ago from down in the corners. (I was much more proficient at keeping the place clean this time around, but I had time on my hands.) I heard something suck-up into the attachment which then stuck in the hose. I shut it off, removed the hose from the vacuum, and tried to beat it out on the carpet, but whatever was in there was stuck. So I got the broom and pushed the handle through the hose until it forced out the obstruction—a wad of dust, crumbs, sunflower seeds, a rubber band, my old dog's fur, paper clips, M&Ms, and a ring. When I removed the ring—an antique, white-gold band with a small diamond setting—I recognized it as Cassidy's, a hand-me-down from her *Granny* that she'd long ago lost and never found. Obviously, it'd fallen down between the cushions of my couch thirty-some years ago. Hmm. She'd probably like to have this back.

I turned on the desktop computer in my home-office, checked my email—mostly junk. Apparently, no one needed my consulting. But of course, I'd neglected to design an ad and purchase ad space. So I went to Facebook instead. I typed in Cassidy's maiden name—I'd heard she married not long after our break-up but had no idea to whom and if she'd changed her name—and a list of similarly-named women and one man's face were thumb-nailed in photos top-to-bottom. I scrolled down the list, but didn't see her. At the bottom, I clicked on "See More Results," and the next face I saw in a thumbnail looked somewhat familiar. But it was the face of a middle-aged woman. I clicked on it. Of course I realized that she, like all of us—except Rose and Al—had aged. But whenever I'd thought of Cassie over the years, it was her sexy-sweet, 25-year-old face that stared back at me. The pink hue was gone from her cheeks, the sparkle from her eyes. And she was wrinkled, like me. I read the most-current post at the top of her public timeline:

"Dear Friends," it started. "As feared, my cancer has metastasized and spread to my other organs. I'll be entering City of Hope next week. I'm on a clinical-trial patient list for CAR-T cell immunotherapy. Hoping I'll qualify. But pancreatic cancer is a tough one to beat—even my oncologist admits we're probably years away from a cure. So if this is to be my last post, thanks for your support & love through these difficult times. Love, Cassidy."

I just sat there for a while—numb—not knowing what to do. I swore a couple times: "God damn cancer!" The post was two-weeks old. I said a prayer for her and closed Facebook.

Over dinner, I mentioned to Anna about Cassidy's condition. They had met briefly one night at the club, during my transition period from one to the other. It had been a little tense as I remembered, working my shift, staying safely behind the bar.

"That's too bad. I hear that's a hard cancer to survive." She nibbled on her salad. "Huh?"

"What?" I washed down my mashed potatoes with a swig of imported beer.

"Why were you looking up your old girlfriend on Facebook?" Her big, brown eyes stared back at me.

"Oh." If I told Anna the truth—that I'd found Cassidy's ring in my old couch and just wanted to return it—I'd be admitting that I'd been back at my old apartment again. And to be honest, I wasn't hurrying to get myself *institutionalized*. "Uh. An old friend e-mailed me. He'd looked her up on Facebook. *Friended* her, I guess. You don't know him." I didn't either because he didn't exist.

She nodded.

There wasn't time to mail the ring as I'd originally planned, so the next morning, I got in my car and drove the 210 Freeway east towards City of Hope. Most of the slow-moving traffic was going the other way towards L.A. (The afternoon would be the reverse.) I got off and parked in their large lot out front that was already mostly-filled with parked cars. As I walked towards the hospital's entrance, I passed a young, slowly-moving couple—she pale with her head wrapped in a scarf; he holding her hand and wearing a pink T-shirt that swore on its front, *"Fu-- Cancer!"*—and crisscrossed paths with other patients—who were easy to spot with their frail appearance and sometimes hairless or cap-covered heads—and their families and friends. It was already getting uncomfortably warm. I was glad I'd worn shorts.

Inside the automatic, double-doors, it was crowded but cool from the air-conditioning. Most of the waiting area's chairs were filled with patients, waiting to hear their names called to have blood drawn, some wearing paper breather-masks to ward-off infection. An older gentleman, clad in a white, dress shirt with neatly-pressed slacks, smiled as he approached me. I guess I looked lost. He wore a button on his chest which read: "VOLUNTEER."

"May I help you, Young Man?"

I smiled, too. No one had referred to me as *Young Man* in a long time. But it was relative. "I'm here to visit a patient friend of mine."

"Let's see if we can find your friend for you. Follow me." He led me to a line at the reception desk, where he waited with me until it was my turn, told the receptionist what I needed, then bid me farewell. "She'll help you from here." He smiled, patted me on the shoulder, then looked to help someone else. I gave the receptionist, seated in front of a computer, Cassidy's name. She told me the wing, floor, and her room number.

There sure were a lot of people sick with cancer. Nurses and doctors walked the wide hallways, too, some of the walls of which were decorated with water-color paintings by the pediatric patients, each signed with a first name, some with an initial, surname tag like: "Alfie T." I was relieved there were no sick kids in this wing. It was hard enough seeing all these sick adults. But sick kids ... it just didn't seem fair. But who said cancer was fair?

I followed the signs to Cassidy's wing of the hospital and took the elevator up to her floor. The nurse at that station gave me a paper breather-mask and a pair of blue, nitrile, examination gloves.

"The patients on this floor have compromised immune systems. So you have to wear these when you visit."

I put on the breather-mask and gloves and followed the room numbers to Cassidy's room, the outside door of which was closed. I looked in through the window in the upper half at an ante-room with a sink. Hand wipes, a box of blue gloves, and masks were on the counter. I went in. The upper half of the interior wall was glass. The curtains inside were pulled back. The woman on the Facebook page—much thinner now, her head bald, her pallor pale, almost gray-like—lay motionless in the hospital bed with an IV needle in her forearm hooked up to an IV drip, looking nothing like the sexy, young woman I'd once dated. A machine kept track of her heartbeats. The TV was on—some talking-heads show—but she didn't appear to be watching. I knocked. When she looked over, I opened the door partially.

"Cassie?"

Her eyes looked tired, with no sign of recognition. But of course, my face was partially-covered with a paper mask and thirty years of wear since she'd last seen it.

"It's Marty."

Her eyebrow-less brow rose and she smiled slightly. "Marty?"

I nodded and walked in. The door closed itself behind me, sealing the room's environment as purified air blew in through its vents. An uneaten meal sat on a tray next to her smartphone.

"Great." Her smile faded. "My ex-boyfriend shows up and I look like hell."

"I'm sorry."

"What are you doing here?"

"I ... uh." I suddenly wasn't sure how to explain. So I reached into my pocket, took out her Granny's ring, and offered it to her in my blue-covered palm.

Her eyes widened and the smile returned as she recognized her ring. "Oh my God." She took it from me, inspecting it closely. "But how?"

"I found it way down below the cushions in the frame of my old couch when I was vacuuming the other day."

She looked at me as if I were crazy. "You still have that same old couch?"

"It's a long story."

"Unfortunately, I don't have time or energy for long stories anymore." She slipped it onto her thin, ring finger, like a wedding band that fit too loosely. "But thanks for my Granny's ring."

"Sure." I nodded. "You're probably tired."

She nodded.

I wasn't sure what to say, how to sign-off. *See you* sure wasn't going to work. So I said: "I'm sorry you're so sick, Cassie."

She smiled a little. "Yeah. Me, too."

I turned to go, but stopped. "Are you getting that cartee cell immunotherapy stuff?"

She didn't look at me, instead, staring at the ring loose on her finger. "Didn't make the cut. Ex-smoker. You know? Dropped me too far down on the list." It was something she had struggled with when we dated; she was always quitting and starting again, quitting and starting again. "That was my last hope to beat this thing." She looked at me, as if for the last time.

So instead of leaving, I pulled up a chair and sat next to her bed. "Maybe not?"

It was like trying to convince someone that an alien spaceship had landed in your back yard. Most folks would think you're nuts. I, too, probably. And so did Cassidy think I had a screw loose when I tried to explain how Al had survived lung cancer for the last 47 years on his side of our stucco-coated, historically-monumental, Fountain-of-Youth duplex. Which meant, of course, that I now had *two* women who thought I needed to be *institutionalized*.

"Look, Marty. I appreciate the ring and it's nice to hear Al's somehow still alive. Rose, too. I always liked her." She paused before continuing, regaining her breath. "But whatever it is, it's not some magical, old house. Magic doesn't cure cancer."

I agreed. "No. But whatever it is that's going on in that old place might keep you alive long enough until this place finds a cure for you."

She scoffed, half-laughing. "Why are you doing this to me? I'm going to die in a week and you come in here with this ridiculous story—" She had run out of breath, started coughing. "Just go, please." She looked away again. "Thanks for my Granny's ring."

So I left. Words weren't going to be enough to convince her. But I had to try. Right? Otherwise...

I'd already tried taking a *selfie* on my smartphone inside my old place as a way to prove to my wife that I was indeed 29 again and wasn't crazy and didn't need to be *institutionalized*. But the photo showed the old me instead. As Rose had said: "It don't work with new folk, Honey." Or new cell-phones. (I couldn't call-out or receive on mine.) So instead, I set-up my smartphone on a step-ladder a few feet away on the front lawn—just out of the duplex's reach—turned on the video-chat and speaker-phone, dialed Cassidy's number, and ran back up on the porch. As her phone rang, the skin on the back of my hands tightened. It rang again. I just hoped this worked and that it was the right number (I'd paid $39.95 to get her cellphone number from PeopleFinders) and that she was in her hospital room—alive. The phone picked up on the other end.

"Hello." Her voice sounded weak over the speaker.

"Hi, Cassie. It's Marty." She didn't say anything, so I continued: "Turn on the video-chat on your phone."

"Why? How'd you get my number?"

"Doesn't matter," I answered. "You don't have to get on-camera yourself. Put your thumb over the lens. But you need to see me."

Again she asked: "Why?"

"Just do it."

There was silence on her end. Assuming she was watching, I smiled and waved, hoping she could see me as myself thirty years ago. I heard a shriek over the speaker-phone— apparently, she could—and the 29-year-old me laughed and said:

"Surpri-i-ise!"

We didn't have much time. The cancer had caused Cassidy's kidneys to shut down. They had given her some drug in an attempt to get them working again. But if that failed, she could go on dialysis tomorrow—*if* she wanted to prolong the inevitable. Her oncologist had told her she only had a few days left. A week at most. Many of her friends and family had already visited for the last time. So we put our plan in motion immediately.

Cassie said there was no way her doctors would cut her loose from the hospital, unless to a hospice or some family member to die at home. So on my way back to City of Hope, I stopped by a hospital supply store, rented a wheelchair, which I folded into my trunk, then stopped at Walmart for some supplies we'd need to make our getaway.

In City of Hope parking lot, I removed the Lakers logo from the lapel button I'd bought at Walmart, wrote "VOL-UNTEER" in block letters on its white backing, and pinned it to the pocket of the white, button-collared, broadcloth shirt I'd worn with long pants. I took the Walmart bag with me, the wheelchair out of the trunk, and rolled into the hospital.

Before I got off the elevator on Cassidy's floor, I put on my own paper breather-mask and nitrile gloves from the Walmart bag. As I rolled the empty wheelchair past the red-headed nurse at her station, I smiled behind my paper mask and nodded. She was busy at her computer, but stopped to give me a look. But she didn't call after me.

I rolled into the ante-room and then into Cassidy's. She glanced over—barely. She looked even weaker than the last time I'd visited.

"You okay?"

"No. I'm dying. Remember? Get my clothes from the closet."

She struggled to sit up in bed and I helped a sick, bald, old lady get dressed—cancer ages you prematurely before it kills you—who in no way resembled the shapely, young woman I'd eagerly helped *un*dress, looking away or closing my eyes as much as possible. It wasn't easy with the IV and heart monitor attached to her finger, which precluded our pulling on the second sleeve of her blouse. If we unhooked it, Cassie said it would sound an alarm and alert the nurses.

I gave her the dark-haired, shoulder-length wig and plastic, over-sized sunglasses from the Walmart bag.

"You couldn't get one with real hair?" She put on the cheap wig, adjusting it in a mirror from her tray. Not satisfied with the artificial hair, she tied a scarf from a drawer around it and put on her own Calvin Klein sunglasses.

"How do I look?"

"Like Jacqueline Kennedy on vacation at Hainesport."

She laughed, then remembered: "She died of cancer, too. You know?"

"You're not going to die. That's why we're doing this."

She took a deep breath and nodded. I helped her into the wheelchair. The IV bottle was on a stand on wheels, so I could roll it along behind her.

"Ready?" I asked.

She took another deep breath and nodded. While I propped the door open with a wastebasket, she put on a breather-mask and one, nitrile glove. I got behind the wheelchair. She breathed haltingly—already tired from dressing—but pulled the heart sensor off her finger. The heart monitor immediately started beeping. I helped her with her sleeve, put a blanket over her lap, then pushed the wheelchair and IV set-up out the opened door, kicking the wastebasket away so it closed behind us. As she put on the other blue glove, we pushed out the second doorway into the hallway. As I rolled Cassidy and her IV bottle down the corridor, another nurse walked quickly past us in the opposite direction. We continued past the red-headed nurse at her station. She again looked up from her computer.

"Excuse me, Sir," she called after us.

I turned my head back but continued pushing the wheelchair. "Just going for a stroll around the wing. Her doctor okayed it."

"Wait a minute. Who is that? Who's her doctor?"

But I didn't look back and didn't stop pushing until we got to the elevators at the end of the hall. I pushed the button. Cassie sat quietly in the wheelchair. I glanced over without making it apparent. The nurse we'd passed in the hallway—headed for Cassidy's room and the beeping heart monitor—was back at the nurses' station now, talking to the red-head behind the computer. They both turned our way. The nurse behind the computer called:

"Sir! You can't take her off this floor!"

The elevator doors opened. I pushed Cassie in the wheelchair with the IV bottle into the already-crowded elevator and turned facing the opened doors, which closed. As the elevator went down towards the ground floor, Cassie's shoulders shook. I leaned over and whispered:

"You okay?"

She nodded behind her sunglasses and breather-mask, under the cheap wig and scarf, trying not to laugh.

But I was paranoid, hoping a siren wouldn't go off, alerting the staff, putting the hospital on lock-down, preventing our escape. Fortunately, there was no siren, no lock-down, and we made our rolling getaway to the parking lot.

The 210 west was backed-up as usual going towards L.A, so I got off the freeway and took Foothill Boulevard back. I tried to drive as fast as I could—Cassie was looking weaker by the mile—without getting stopped for speeding.

I didn't want to explain to a cop what a half-dead woman wrapped in a blanket, hooked up to an IV bottle was doing in my car and why we were both wearing masks and blue, examination gloves. Half-an-hour later, I pulled into the driveway and drove all the way to the front of the duplex. I turned off the engine. Her breathing came haltingly, her head down.

"We're here, Cassie."

She looked up, but didn't say anything.

I got out and quickly removed and unfolded the wheel-chair from the trunk. But when I rolled it to the passenger side and opened the door, Cassie's head was down on her chest again—the sunglasses had fallen from her face—and only the seatbelt was holding her up. I wasn't sure if she was still breathing behind the paper mask.

"Cassie? You okay?"

She didn't answer. I unhooked the IV bag from its metal support collapsed in the back seat, unbuckled Cassidy and struggled to lift her—she didn't weigh much now but I wasn't as strong as I used to be either—out of the car with the IV bag on her lap.

"Cassie!"

She lay limply in my arms, head back, and didn't answer.

"Damnit!"

Instead of putting her in the wheelchair, I carried her in my arms hurriedly across the yard and up the steps onto the front porch. As I began to feel stronger, I felt her breathing again in my arms. The wrinkles disappeared from her brow and her eyebrows sprouted. Her breasts firmed under her

115

blouse. She lifted her head, batted her baby-blue eyes, and stared into mine. She pulled off her mask and the wig and scarf; her silky, dark hair grew back. Her alabaster skin was smooth and the rosy hue returned to her cheeks. Then she removed my mask and smiled at the 29-year-old me, still holding her in my muscular arms like some young stud on the cover of a romance novel.

"Do I look like you?" she asked.

"Better," I admitted.

She smiled and with her blue-gloved hand, pulled the IV needle out of her arm, leaving only a drop of blood on her smooth, white skin.

I smiled, too. "Welcome back."

"Where were you?" Anna asked when I got home that evening.

I'd stayed at my old house with Cassie longer than I should have. But how could I not? There had been lots to explain; that that I could. "Uh, you know." I pretended to swing a golf club.

"Don't you need your clubs to play golf?"

Uh oh. I'd taken them out of the trunk of my car to accommodate the wheelchair and had left them in the garage. "Oh, I, uh, borrowed a friend's instead. He got some new clubs. I might buy his old ones."

"Really?" She didn't seem convinced. She sighed, as if blowing out candles on a birthday cake. "You've been going back there again. Haven't you?"

I didn't answer at first. But she already knew.

Cassie and I had broken up long ago when I found out that I was likewise her *main squeeze*. We'd both slept around outside our relationship—I with a series of one-night-stands after closing-time; she with her Ex, the same damn guy I'd thrown out of the club! Not that we'd ever agreed to be faithful to one another. We'd both carefully sidestepped that issue. I'd just assumed she was even though I wasn't. And I couldn't handle it when I found out otherwise. My bad, I guess. Lesson learned. I parked out front and walked down the driveway with a bag of groceries. Rose, in her usual attire, stood on the porch like a sentry, watering the flowers and shrubs out front with a hose. Because they couldn't leave the duplex, she had their groceries and Al's cigarettes delivered once a week to the front porch.

"Afternoon, Honey."

For some reason, I felt as if I'd been *busted*. "Oh, hi, Rose." I stepped up on the porch and became 29 again as I pulled open the screen door.

"What's your rush?"

Al started hacking somewhere inside their apartment.

"Uh, no, no rush." I turned back to her. "What's up?"

"Leopard don't change its spots much. Do it, Honey?" She gave me a side-long glance—apparently aware my old girlfriend was inside—as she watered the little flowers. She'd been an eyewitness to my revolving-girlfriend policy of the past.

"What?" I wanted to explain how I was innocent of any misdeeds and that having my ex-girlfriend now living inside my old apartment was actually a benevolent act on my part, not some horn-dog maneuver to get laid. But the circumstantial evidence was damning in itself. What would Anna say? I hadn't figured that one out yet either. The Hulk-green front door suddenly opened partially from inside and Cassie peeked out. She batted her baby-blues and smiled her sexy-sweet, 25-year-old smile and my knees went weak. I really hadn't thought through the ramifications of this whole scenario. So I didn't inquire further of Rose about her big cat metaphor; I knew what she meant.

"See you later."

"Yeah," Rose said, before I went inside. "See ya', Honey."

I closed the door behind.

Cassidy liked being young and beautiful again, too. She had married the same ex-boyfriend that I'd thrown out of the club but they were divorced now. Had been for years. Their daughter lived on the east coast. Cassie had a boy-friend. And because I was still married, she wanted to invite him over. But I told her it didn't work with *new folk*, as Rose had pointed out, and that she'd risk turning back into a sickly, old lady with cancer again if he entered the duplex. That freaked her out.

"So I can't leave? And you're the only one who can come inside."

"Sorry. Not my rules."

"Oh." The ramifications likewise took her aback. "And my iPhone's dead," she said, as if eulogizing a best friend.

Cassidy wanted me to go back to her apartment and get some of her things. But if I got caught, there'd be no way to explain my being there. Besides, her clothes wouldn't fit her 25-year-old-bod now anyway. So as per her precise instructions, I bought her a few outfits at the mall. (I always wore different shirts and pants to my old place, so apparently clothing—like food—wasn't a problem. Re-live and learn.) It was weird shopping in the ladies departments—especially buying undergarments. The salesgirl gave me a weird look. I didn't try to explain. I paid and got the heck out of there.

Cassie looked good in her new clothes, one cleavage-baring top in particular. It was hard not to stare, and before I went back to my real life, we almost kissed goodbye on the porch, standing close, staring into each other's young eyes again. It was all I could do to walk away. But I was still married.

"You playing golf again Saturday?" Anna asked. She was correcting papers as usual on the dining room table.

I'd been pretending to play regularly on Saturday afternoons. "Two-o'clock tee time, as usual." I smiled back. More lies.

"Did you ever take that lesson?"

"No, I never did. But I sure need one. I swing like a chicken with its head cut off." I wasn't sure that was the best simile, but it somehow seemed appropriate.

She half-laughed. "I'd like to see that."

"No, I don't think you would."

Saturday afternoon, I put on my golf shirt. The clubs were already in the trunk. (I double-checked.) Anna had already left for the supermarket and her weekly shopping.

She'd be gone for hours, too. I parked around the block from Poppy Way—in case Anna drove by so she wouldn't see my car—and walked the rest of the way. I needed a new plan. If I kept going back to the old place, it was only a matter of time before I gave in to lust. I'd been infatuated with Cassie once before. And she was great in bed. I half-laughed. Except, of course, for our last night together, when she'd confessed to boinking her ex-boyfriend again. So I couldn't take the chance. Anna already thought I was nuts. I couldn't be unfaithful, too. She'd divorce me. Rose's *leopard spots* had been a warning. She knew me well. But a cop car was parked out front at the curb and when I turned down the driveway, the same young cop—this time wearing sunglasses, like me—walked up the driveway away from the old duplex.

"What are you doing here again?" he asked.

"That's what I was going to ask you, Officer."

"Report of someone around back again. Didn't see any sign of a break-in. Now you."

"Just stopped by to visit Rose and Al. My old neighbors," I explained.

"They're not here. I knocked."

"I'll leave a note."

He eyed me from behind his shades.

I returned a smile and continued to the back. He went the other way. I waited near the porch, until I saw his patrol car drive past at the end of the driveway, then stepped up. As I un-aged, I heard Rose laughing inside her side of the duplex with someone else. Who, I wondered? I opened the screen door on my side and knocked. I didn't know what to do? What would happen? I couldn't cheat on Anna. But of course, behind that Hulk-green door, inside my old place with Cassidy was actually *before* I'd met Anna. So technically, it wouldn't be cheating. Aw hell, I was just rationalizing. I knew it. I was acting 29 again, too—a *leopard's spots*. I knocked again. When Cassie didn't answer, I tried the knob—the key was around back if I needed it—but the door was unlocked.

Inside, the turntable was already turning and Roberta Flack sang: "*Strumming my pain with his fingers, Singing my life with his words. Killing me softly...*" Uh oh. I gulped. The hallway was always dark even in the daytime. I followed it to the bedroom doorway. I took a deep breath, pushed open the partially-closed door, and walked in.

"Surpri-i-ise!"

And there under the top-sheet of my waterbed, lay my beautiful, 24-year-old, future bride, smiling back at me as she hadn't smiled at me in a long time. The front door key lay atop the nearby nightstand.

"I changed my mind, Hon." Anna slowly pulled back the sheet, inviting me in.

I bought a new set of golf clubs and took a few lessons, but I still swung like a chicken with its head cut off. But at least I didn't have to lie anymore as to my whereabouts to Anna. She and Cassidy had talked that afternoon before my arrival, so she knew the whole story now. And I convinced the ladies, *let's-not-look-a-gift-horse-in-the-mouth* was our best approach to the inexplicable. So we all stopped trying to figure it out. Why take a chance of breaking *the spell*, and in the process, killing two cancer patients and Rose? Sometimes there was no guide book and you had to figure things out for yourselves. I retired my consulting business. Because Anna and I didn't want to outlive our kids, we decided to grow old together and die naturally, unlike Rose and Al, who had opted for the thin plaster walls and peeling stucco exterior of immortality—Who knew how long they'd survive? As long as the old duplex stood?—and Cassidy, who waited impatiently, alluringly for a cure. Anna and I only visited our Fountain of Youth once a week on Saturday nights—like a tryst with smooth skin and firm flesh—while Cassie had dinner with Rose and a cigarette with Al in the apartment next door. We kept a low profile just the same, so the cops wouldn't keep snooping about. (There had been a blurb in the *L.A. Times* and a short segment on a local newscast about our escape from City of Hope—a video-camera had recorded our exit as we passed its lens, but my face was looking down and unidentifiable—and Cassidy's subsequent disappearance.) I put the key on a silver chain around my neck and wore it like a Saint Christopher medal, patron saint of travelers. As Rose had warned, making a copy and trying it in the lock would be risky. Some things you just knew. And I couldn't take a chance on the key disappearing now if someone from the electric company stopped by to read the meter and happened upon it. Ponce de Leon would've been proud. It was a workable lesson plan. At least for now. And maybe even—for eternity?

HAPPY BIRTHDAY

Saturday, June 6th, 2015 was my birthday. I was four-years old. Admittedly, not as cute as most four-year-olds. But surely, a lot luckier than most. That's because four years ago, I got a stem cell transplant at City of Hope that saved my life. As the nurse hung the IV bag with my recondi-tioned stem cells, she said to me:

"Congratulations, today is your new birthday."

As usual, I woke early. While sipping cups of strong, black coffee and consuming Nature Valley granola bars, I did a few hours work in my garage-office. After which, I fed the dogs, chugged down a fruit smoothie with a handful of vitamins and my meds, then hopped on my mountain bike to scale the inclined streets of Sierra Bonita Avenue up to its northern boundary at William Carey International Univer-sity. I zigged and zagged upon the weaving walkways of the theological campus—more aggressively than I should have, considering I'd crashed recently, going too fast (x-rays on my right shoulder inconclusive, MRI still pending)—until the campus security guard showed up in his three-wheeler.

I jockeyed back out onto the streets and sidewalks, up-and-down driveways, over to Sandwiches by Connal's for a late breakfast-to-go, which I tied to my handlebars, like a little kid returning with a plastic bagful of goodies from the store. At home, I brunched on a scrumptious BLT-with-scrambled-eggs-on-toast in front of the TV, where the best skateboarders in the world annihilated a skate park at the X-Games in Austin, Texas, then turned on the DVR to watch Serena Williams win the French Open on the red clay courts of Roland Garros. I perused the *L.A. Times* Sports page (best in the west), called my Mom (88 and hanging in there), and bench-pressed (at a reduced-weight due to my injured shoulder, bandaged with kinesiology tape) in the garage. I watched on TV as American Pharoah won the Triple Crown of horse-racing at the Belmont Stakes in New York, completing my video tour. I took a rejuvenating power-nap (I loved naps!), walked and fed the dogs dinner, then showered and shaved and headed off to California Pizza Kitchen with my lovely wife to celebrate. I toasted the doctors, nurses, family, friends, and Big Guy &/or Gal upstairs who helped save my life:

"Thanks, All! I'd be dead without you!" That platinum margarita—silver *Patron* tequila splashed with *Grand Mariner* liqueur and lime juice, on the rocks, garnished with a lime wedge and salted rim—sure tasted mighty good!

CHECK-UP

Along with the medical diagrams and charts and posters about clinical trials on the walls of the examination room at the Alhambra office of UCLA Hematology & Oncology Health, was a book laid opened to a Biblical quote of the day. I always read them while I waited for my oncologist Dr. Hu to step in. I wasn't a true *believer*—but I was a true *hoper*. I had daily conversations with Whoever or Whatever was on the *other side*—*if* there were another side. I found it comforting to think so. I imagined being again with those who'd passed before me—family, friends, my old dogs—in a peaceful setting. After all, there was no *getting-out alive*. So I tried not to be anxious as I waited. Sure, I knew a bad report would mean I was back in treatment—heavy treatment—unlike the 21-pills-a-month-with-no-side-effects I now took to keep the cancer from returning. But when those thoughts arose, I fought back with my mantra: *I don't have cancer and it's not coming back!* I sure as heck wasn't going to waste the good times I had left worrying about the bad times that might befall me again someday. That seemed counter-

125

productive to my happy life.

"Hmm," Dr. Hu mused, reading my most-recent blood-work chart on the computer. "Your M-spike is gone." The *M-spike* was a mark on my kidneys that meant multiple myeloma—the incurable cancer which had been jettisoned from my blood and bones with chemo and a stem cell transplant—was still in my system. Dormant—but still there.

"I thought you said that wouldn't happen?"

"It usually doesn't."

"Huh?" I smiled, pounded my heart twice with my fist, and offered a peace sign to the heavens. "Imagine that."

CREDITS

"Better Boobs," *Notes Magazine*, Literature Finalist, Issue #5, Grace Notes Publishing, San Bernardino, CA, '12; *And We Write: Surviving Cancer; Let the Healing Begin*, Wheatmark Publishing, Tucson, AZ, '11; www.chicklitreview.org, March/April Issue, Fiction section, '09; www.farmhousemagazine.com, March/April Issue, Fiction section, '08; *Illness & Grace, Terror & Transformation*, Wising Up Press, GA, '07; www.voidmagazine.com, Sept. Issue, Fiction section, '06; www.girlswithinsurance.com, Feb Issue, Fiction section, '05.

"Marathon Man," www.thewriteplaceatthewritetime.org, *Our Stories* Section, Winter/Spring Issue, '15.

"A Pretty Good Deal," *High Hopes*, Vol. 9, City of Hope Family Resource Center, Fall Issue, '13; www.thewriteplaceatthewritetime.org, Poetry Section, Autumn Issue, '11.

"Sick as a Dog," *High Hopes*, Vol. 10, City of Hope Family
Resource Center, Winter Issue, '15;
www.commonlinejournal.com, Issue #18, Fall, '12; *Line
Zero*, Literature Finalist, Vol. 2, Issue 3, Pink Fish Press,
6/'12.

"*Electrified!*" www.chimaeraserials.com, Premiere Issue,
8/'06.

"Amphibious Again,"
www.thewriteplaceatthewritetime.org, *Our Stories* Section, Summer Issue, '15.

Back Cover Photo
by
Dan Unfried

Woof dog
by
Jolly John Rogers

When you buy this book,
you contribute to City of Hope
and their fight against cancer.

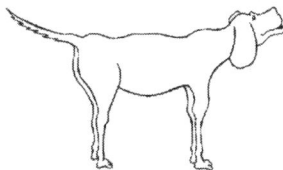

WOOF BOOKS

San Marino, CA

www.markbark.org

Made in the USA
San Bernardino, CA
15 October 2015